Healing
Life's Crises

D1227647

Healing
Life's Crises
A Guide for Nurses

NOREEN CAVAN FRISCH, PhD, RN
Professor and Chair
Department of Nursing
Humboldt State University
Arcata, California

JANE KELLEY, PhD, RN
Professor
Department of Nursing
Southeast Missouri State University
Cape Girardeau, Missouri

Delmar Publishers

 I(T)P™

An International Thomson Publishing Company

Albany • Bonn • Boston • Cincinnati • Detroit • London
Madrid • Melbourne • Mexico City • New York • Pacific Grove
Paris • San Francisco • Singapore • Tokyo • Toronto • Washington

NOTICE TO THE READER

Publisher does not warrant or guarantee any of the products described herein or perform any independent analysis in connection with any of the product information contained herein. Publisher does not assume, and expressly disclaims, any obligation to obtain and include information other than that provided to it by the manufacturer.

The reader is expressly warned to consider and adopt all safety precautions that might be indicated by the activities herein and to avoid all potential hazards. By following the instructions contained herein, the reader willingly assumes all risks in connection with such instructions.

The publisher makes no representation or warranties of any kind, including but not limited to, the warranties of fitness for particular purpose or merchantability, nor are any such representations implied with respect to the material set forth herein, and the publisher takes no responsibility with respect to such material. The publisher shall not be liable for any special, consequential, or exemplary damages resulting, in whole or part, from the readers' use of, or reliance upon, this material.

Cover Design: Spiral Design
Cover Illustration: Kirsten Soderlind

Delmar Staff
Publisher: Diane L. McOscar
Senior Acquisitions Editor: Bill Burgower
Assistant Editor: Debra M. Flis
Project Editor: Judith Boyd Nelson
Production Coordinator: Barbara A. Bullock
Art and Design Coordinator: Mary E. Siener
Editorial Assistant: Chrisoula Baikos

COPYRIGHT © 1996
By Delmar Publishers
a division of International Thomson Publishing Inc.

The ITP logo is a trademark under license.

Printed in the United States of America

For more information, contact:

Delmar Publishers
3 Columbia Circle, Box 15015
Albany, New York 12212-5015

International Thomson Publishing Europe
Berkshire House 168-173
High Holborn
London, WC1V 7AA
England

Thomas Nelson Australia
102 Dodds Street
South Melbourne, 3205
Victoria, Australia

Nelson Canada
1120 Birchmont Road
Scarborough, Ontario
Canada, M1K 5G4

International Thomson Editores
Campos Eliseos 385, Piso 7
Col Polanco
11560 Mexico D F Mexico

International Thomson Publishing GmbH
Konigswinterer Strasse 418
53227 Bonn
Germany

International Thomson Publishing Asia
221 Henderson Road
#05-10 Henderson Building
Singapore 0315

International Thomson Publishing—Japan
Hirakawacho Kyowa Building, 3F
2-2-1 Hirakawacho
Chiyoda-ku, Tokyo 102
Japan

All rights reserved. No part of this work covered by the copyright hereon may be reproduced or used in any form or by any means — graphic, electronic, or mechanical, including photocopying, recording, taping, or information storage and retrieval systems — without the written permission of the publisher.

1 2 3 4 5 6 7 8 9 10 XXX 01 00 99 98 97 96 95

Library of Congress Cataloging-in-Publication Data

Frisch, Noreen Cavan.
    Healing life's crises: a guide for nurses /
Noreen Cavan Frisch. Jane Kelley. — 1st ed.
        p.   cm. — (Nurse as healer series)
    Includes bibliographical references and index.
    ISBN 0-8273-6399-0
    1. Nursing—Psychological aspects.   2. Crisis intervention
(Psychiatry)   3. Nurse and patient.   4. Life change events.
I. Kelley, Jane, 1944–   . II. Title. III. Series.
RT86.F75   1996
610.73 — dc20
                                                      94–48614
                                                      CIP

INTRODUCTION TO NURSE AS HEALER SERIES

LYNN KEEGAN, PhD, RN, Series Editor

*Associate Professor, School of Nursing,
University of Texas Health Science Center at San Antonio
and Director of BodyMind Systems, Temple, TX*

To nurse means to care for or to nurture with compassion. Most nurses begin their formal education with this ideal. Many nurses retain this orientation after graduation, and some manage their entire careers under this guiding principle of caring. Many of us, however, tend to forget this ideal in the hectic pace of our professional and personal lives. We may become discouraged and feel a sense of burnout.

Throughout the past decade I have spoken at many conferences with thousands of nurses. Their experience of frustration and failure is quite common. These nurses feel themselves spread as pawns across a health care system too large to control or understand. In part, this may be because they have forgotten their true roles as nurse-healers.

When individuals redirect their personal vision and empower themselves, an entire pattern may begin to change. And so it is now with the nursing profession. Most of us conceptualize nursing as much more than a vocation. We are greater than our individual roles as scientists, specialists, or care deliverers. We currently search for a name to put on our new conception of the empowered nurse. The recently introduced term *nurse-healer* aptly describes the qualities of an increasing number of clinicians, educators, administrators, and nurse practitioners. Today all nurses are awakening to the realization that they have the potential for healing.

It is my feeling that most nurses, when awakened and guided to develop their own healing potential, will function both as nurses and healers. Thus, the concept of nurse as healer is born. When nurses realize they have the ability to evoke others' healing, as well as care for them, a shift of consciousness begins to occur. As individual awareness and changes in skill building occur, a collective understanding of this new concept emerges. This knowledge, along with a shift in attitudes and new kinds of behavior, allows empowered nurses to renew themselves in an expanded role. The Nurse As Healer Series is born out of the belief that nurses are ready to embrace guidance that inspires them in their journeys of empowerment. Each book in the series may stand alone or be used in complementary fashion with other books. I hope and believe that information herein will strengthen you both personally and professionally, and provide you with the help and confidence to embark upon the path of nurse-healer.

Titles in the Nurse As Healer Series:

Healing Touch: A Resource for Health Care Professionals

Healing Life's Crises: A Guide for Nurses

The Nurse's Meditative Journal

Healing Nutrition

Healing the Dying

Awareness in Healing

Creative Imagery in Nursing

DEDICATION

*The authors dedicate this work to
Linda Hunter, MSN, RN, who shared her work,
life, and friendship with us while she taught us
how to live life and approach death.*

C O N T E N T S

PREFACE

As part of the Nurse As Healer series, this book provides the practicing nurse with a new look at the concept of "crisis intervention." In the literature, crisis intervention is used to describe the nursing/health care responses to clients in some kind of emergency situation. Typically, nurses think of crises as those situations requiring immediate counseling, usually counseling of a short-term nature. Nurses involved in crisis hotlines provide support to those under stress resulting from assault and trauma, physical abuse, depression, and suicidal ideation. Nurses on crisis teams in the community respond to calls from distressed families and individuals. Nurses in emergency departments become skilled in handling the anxieties and stress associated with accidents and injuries. In acute care settings, nurses care for clients undergoing treatment for numerous medical conditions resulting in an upset or upheaval of the person's life. Thus, nurses see these situations as the unusual events in an individual's life, the unexpected situations that leave the clients and their families coping with unanticipated consequences.

Although most nurses have developed the skills in helping clients cope with crises, a nurse as *healer* will go beyond the immediate crisis or precipitating event to understand the crisis event in terms of the whole client. For years, nurses have observed that a crisis is in the eye of the beholder: that is, a particular situation will be a crisis for one individual and not for another. Starting from this observation, we will examine the crisis as a natural event of living as well as an unusual one. We will consider which skills for living aid one in facing the inevitable, unpredictable, and critical occurrences that change the course of one's life, work, and/or relationships. From this perspective, nurses are invited to explore the meanings of living, growing, and changing as we look in-depth at individuals' efforts to order, control, and make sense of their experiences.

This book is organized into four parts: an introduction to the meaning of a crisis as a challenge; an evaluation of crisis in relation to body, mind, and spirit; a look at special client situations; and lastly, an examination of specific tools for dealing with crises.

Chapter 1 introduces the idea of a crisis as a challenge and explores the various ways in which crisis presents and affects the person as a whole. The Modeling and Role-Modeling nursing theory is introduced as a basis for holistic nursing care. Chapter 2 examines the challenges of physical illness. Through understanding of the experience of illness, nurses are assisted in facilitating successful resolution of crisis events for their clients. Chapter 3 examines situations where persons perceive mental anguish and evaluate the subjective experiences of such events. From the understanding gleaned, the authors consider nursing interventions useful to assist clients dealing mentally with difficult situations and events. Chapter 4 provides nurses with a picture of how to identify and care for a client experiencing a spiritual crisis. Issues addressed include: What constitutes the spiritual component of a person? How is the spiritual component related to health? When is there evidence of a spiritual crisis? What is the nursing role in spiritual care? Chapter 5 addresses the special situation of the client who is dying. This chapter explores the role of caregivers in assisting dying clients through the crisis of dying, employing techniques of healing rather than of curing. Chapter 6 focuses on the special considerations of the client facing a significant loss. The definitions of grieving and the subjective experience of grief are presented, along with suggestions for appropriate and sensitive interventions. Chapter 7 examines families from a perspective of family theory and family development, as well as from nursing theory. Nurses are frequently called upon to assist families facing crises. Approaches for assessment and interventions are presented. To address tools for preventing crises in nurses' lives, chapter 8 evaluates organizations from the perspective of nursing theory and discusses how organizations work and what can be done to affect positive change. Chapter 9 provides information on conflict resolution. Written by Mr. Evan Ferber, Executive Director of the Dispute Resolution Center of Thurston Co., Olympia, WA, this chapter examines interpersonal and multiparty conflict as stressors that contribute to disease. Practical working models of community-based conflict resolution are introduced for nurses to use in their own self-care, as well as referral sources for clients.

Throughout the book, the authors recognize that life's challenges produce crises for individuals and groups. We believe that positive nursing interventions can help to heal and can assist others in finding peace and health in their lives.

A C K N O W L E D G M E N T S

The authors wish to acknowledge our teachers, students, and colleagues who have helped us understand the holism of nursing. Particularly, we thank Dr. Helen Erickson, whose work and enthusiasm for nursing have provided great motivation, and Professor Marshelle Thobaben for her assistance in the review of this manuscript. We thank Bob Boden, RN, who assisted with the graphics. We also thank Stephanie Ericsson for publishing her personal account of grief, which provided us the ability to learn and, ultimately, to support others.

Lastly, we acknowledge the dual muses of Art and Music who provide lasting inspiration for our lives.

CRISIS, A DEFINITION AND NEW UNDERSTANDING

1 THE CRISIS AS ONE OF LIFE'S CHALLENGES

Nurses are often called upon to deal with crises. In any given day, a nurse may face crisis in the staffing schedule, crisis for the patient with a disturbing diagnosis, crisis for the family victimized by assault, crisis for the teenager suffering from an accident, or crisis for the patient contemplating suicide. These examples are typical of the crises encountered at work. In addition to these, of course, nurses will face their own individual crises, such as failed babysitting arrangements, cars that do not work, minor health problems, and the inability to complete a day's work in a day. Further, as members of society, nurses are constantly reminded of crisis situations around the world—crises of the environment, the economy, and politics of the world. Nurses may rightly feel that enough is enough and that they cannot be responsible for resolving all of the crises that surround them. Indeed, nurses may find that dealing with their own crises leaves them with little energy or interest left to devote to uncovering additional crises from patients or others.

To experience crisis is to experience anxiety. A crisis is an unexpected situation that upsets a plan. As such, a crisis leaves a person out of control, often in a state of powerlessness. A crisis may leave one angry as well, for when something doesn't work out as it should, a person may ask, "Why me?" "Why today?" "What did I do to deserve this?" To understand and cope with crisis, one must understand these feelings of anxiety, anger and powerlessness. Further, one must appreciate the relationship of crisis to day-to-day living. Although nurses recognize that living means growing and changing, developing new ideas, thoughts, and attitudes, they have had little help in incorporating these ideas into their living and their practice.

WHAT IS CRISIS?

Is a crisis always a bad thing? Common usage provides the connotation that it is. No one would wish for a crisis. No one would ask to be out of control or to have an unexpected demand placed on them. Let us begin by searching definitions of the word *crisis* and determine the actual meaning of the word.

Definitions and Kinds of Crises

The *Oxford English Dictionary* (1971, p. 1178) defines crisis as the "turning point in a disease . . . the decisive stage in the progress of anything, a state of affairs in which change for the better or worse is imminent." The original usage of the term was the turning point of an illness. The *Webster's New World Dictionary* (1982, p. 336) defines a crisis as a "turning point," or a "decisive or crucial time, stage, or event." Nursing literature defines crisis in various ways: as an "upset in a steady state" (Baird, 1976, p. 37); "an internal disturbance that results from a stressful event or perceived threat to self" (Stuart & Sundeen, 1991, p. 272); "an experience of being confronted with an unfamiliar obstacle in life's path" (Cunningham, 1991, p. 760); and a "situation that exists when coping responses to stress fail, and the event is experienced as overwhelming" (Berger & Williams, 1992, p. G-4).

There is general agreement that there are two kinds of crises: *situational*—those events that pose a threat to the individual's steady state, and *maturational*—the stressors associated with the individual's moving through life's stages and roles. Some writers suggest that maturational crises are common, normal, and positive and that situational crises are uncommon, unusual, and negative. This assignment of crises into simple categories may be useful to describe how one can differentiate between situations that are more or less predictable and those that seem random. For many individuals, however, the subjective experience of crises is the same regardless of the categorization used. For example, the movement in social roles from married woman to widow is a predictable, maturational change that will occur for many women. Experience with women undergoing these adjustments, however, indicates that the incident is unwanted, painful, and anything but positive. Therefore, it may be best for nurses to use a simple definition of the term *crisis*—a turning point, a situation causing an unexpected change in life—and leave it to the client to fill in the rest as an individual expression of the actual, subjective experience of the crisis event.

Crises versus Challenges

Although the experience of coping with a crisis is unpleasant, the actual resolution of a crisis may not be a bad thing at all. Let's return to the example of women moving from the role of wife to widow. These women never wished to go through the experience of the death of a spouse, yet many women will describe the positive aspects of a rediscovery of self after such a change. Similarly, some patients with significant, life-threatening illnesses, such as cancer, may describe coping with the illness as a constructive experience that positively changed their lives (Fryback, 1993). These views have led the authors to take the approach that all crises can and should be viewed in terms of challenges. Simply defined, a *challenge* is anything that calls for special effort or dedication. Clearly, to rise to the challenge of a maturational change, to deal with the experience of a life-threatening illness, or to meet the unexpected in day-to-day life is to apply the special effort or dedication necessary to managing one's life and emerging as a whole and healthy being. Nursing has a role in assisting clients to learn to cope with challenges in ways that support growth, development, and health. To accomplish meeting life's challenges in this manner, nurses must understand themselves and their clients from a holistic perspective.

A HOLISTIC VIEW OF THE PERSON

The word *holistic* has been used for some time in nursing writings. The major notion behind the concept is that the person is understood as more than a biological, physical body that presents with some clinical condition requiring care. Nurses have identified that they provide care to the whole person, taking responsibility for supporting their clients' physical, emotional, mental, and spiritual states.

Two Views

The term *holistic* has acquired two quite distinct meanings in the nursing literature. One view is that the person is understood as having various components, that is, biophysical, psychological, and spiritual, which together make the whole. The whole is understood to be greater than the sum of the parts. This school of thought permits nurses to think of the person in segments. For example, a nurse may assess the person's emotional state and separate it from the person's physical condition. This allows nurses to talk about a patient's positive outlook, such as his emotions of cheer in spite of a physical diagnosis of cancer. Such a framework permits nurses to assess various aspects of individuals and put together an entire picture of the person's state of well-being. Figure 1.1 illustrates this view, depicting the interpenetration of the energies of the person.

Under the second emerging view of the holistic concept, the person is understood to mean *the whole*—the being in its entirety. Grounded in the nursing theories of Rogers (Falco & Lobo, 1990) and Newman (Cross, 1993), this view suggests that it is impossible to divide the person into components and maintain an understanding of the whole. Persons are whole entities, and our assessments and language must reflect wholism. Thus, describing a person as a "unitary human being" and acknowledging the human energy field as an irreducible unit is a Rogerian interpretation of holistic.

In 1992, the American Holistic Nurses Association (AHNA) presented a description of holistic nursing that addresses both of these views. The AHNA description is given following figure 1.1.

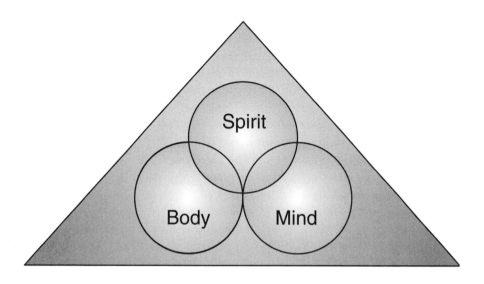

FIGURE 1.1 Components of the person and the interpenetration of the energies of the person.

The Description of Holistic Nursing

Holistic nursing embraces all nursing practice which has the health of the whole person as its goal. Holistic nursing recognizes that there are two views regarding holism: that holism involves studying and understanding the interrelationships of the bio-psycho-social-spiritual dimensions of the person, recognizing that the whole is greater than the sum of its parts; and that holism involves understanding the individual as an integrated whole interacting with and being acted upon by both internal and external environments. Holistic nursing accepts both views, believing that the goals of nursing can be achieved within either framework.

Holistic practice draws on nursing knowledge, theories, expertise, and intuition to guide nurses in becoming therapeutic partners with clients in strengthening the clients' responses to facilitate the healing process and achieve wholeness.

Practicing holistic nursing requires nurses to integrate self-care in their own lives. Self-responsibility leads the nurse to a greater awareness of the interconnectedness of all individuals and their relationships to the human and global community, and permits nurses to use this awareness to facilitate healing. (American Holistic Nurses Association, 1992, used with permission.)

Inherent in this description is the notion that holistic nurses can and do work within both frameworks. The basic definition of holistic care is that the nurse provides care to the whole person. Nurses themselves must choose the theories that support their practice and the terminology and language that assist them in understanding and describing their care.

For the purposes of this book, the definition of the person as having various components—physical, emotional, mental, and spiritual is used. We believe that any factor affecting one component will have a direct and immediate effect on the others. Further, we believe that the person is greater than the sum of the components and that these components are used as a means of clarifying and teaching what we experience. We do not discount the view that the person can be understood in terms of the totality, for example, in terms of the unitary human being. However, we have found the ability to describe various components useful. For this reason, we examine the various crises or challenges that individuals encounter as challenges of the physical, emotional, mental, or spiritual realm.

GOALS OF THE HOLISTIC NURSE

To appreciate the person as holistic, one must also acknowledge the individual as having a past and a future, and as moving through time on her own life's journey. Nurse theorist Helen Erickson states that a nurse's encounter with a patient is like opening up a book to the middle pages. Nurses must understand there is always something that went on before and something that will go on after their professional encounter with any client (Erickson, Tomlin, & Swain, 1983). Each person is moving through life, facing physical changes, emotional events, developmental tasks, and dealing with uncertainty. Individuals have their own personalities which permit varying degrees of flexibility or rigidity. Further, individuals have various repertoires of coping behaviors to call upon when encountering new and challenging situations. An individual is not static, but rather a developing, changing being affected by his past, dealing with the present. A nurse's goals are to understand the client as an individual, to provide empathy and support for the client facing challenges, to enhance the client's movement through developmental and/or maturational changes, and to assist the client in learning to cope. Professional nurses find that use of a nursing theory to guide practice assists in accomplishing these goals. The authors have chosen the Modeling and Role-Modeling theory as the framework to use in understanding the client holistically and to guide practice in crisis-producing and challenging situations.

THE MODELING AND ROLE-MODELING THEORY

The description of this theory is taken from a summary of Modeling and Role-Modeling developed by Frisch and Bowman (1995, used with permission). First published in the book *Modeling and Role-Modeling: a Theory and Paradigm for Nursing* (Erickson et al., 1983), the Modeling and Role-Modeling theory represents a holistic framework for nursing that is heavily grounded in theories of psychosocial development. Since the original publication, research and theory development continues through the efforts of many nurses and the Society for the Advancement of Modeling and Role-Modeling.

The theory is an interpersonal and interactive theory of nursing that requires the nurse to assess (model), plan (role-model), and intervene (five aims of intervention) based on the client's perspective of the world. The nurse always acknowledges the uniqueness and individuality of the client and appreciates that individuals, at some level, know what makes them ill and what makes them well (self-care knowledge). Two additional concepts important in this theory are: (1) affiliated-individuation, and (2) adaptive potential.

Modeling

Modeling is both an art and a science. It is the process used by the nurse when developing an understanding of the client's world as the client perceives it. The way an individual perceives life and all of its aspects and components; the way an individual thinks, communicates, feels, believes, and behaves; and the underlying motivation and rationale for beliefs and behaviors all comprise the individual's model of the world. The art of modeling is the empathetic development of an understanding of the present situation within the client's context of the world; that is, the development of a *model* of the situation from the client's perspective. The science of modeling is the analysis of the information collected about the client's world. The client's perspective is analyzed on the basis of knowledge and theory regarding human behavior, development, cultural diversity, interaction, pathophysiology, human needs, and so on (Erickson et al., 1983).

Role-Modeling

Role-modeling is the facilitation of health. It is also both an art and a science. The art of role-modeling involves the individualization of care based on the client's model of the world; the science of role-modeling is the utilization of theoretical bases when planning and implementing nursing care. Role-modeling is the facilitation of the individual in attaining, maintaining, or promoting health through purposeful interventions that are based on the individual's personal perceptions as well as the theoretical base for the practice of nursing.

Interventions

The aims of intervention are based on five principles pertaining to similarities among humans. Because each individual is unique and has his own model of the world, standardized interventions are not possible to formulate. However, since all humans have some similarities, the aims of intervention can be standardized. Individualized interventions are based on the client's model of the world and are guided by the five aims of intervention as defined here:

1. *Build trust.* Nursing requires a trusting relationship between nurse and client. This relationship involves honesty, acceptance, respect, empathy, and a belief in the client's model of the world.

2. *Promote positive orientation.* Nursing interventions need to promote self-worth as well as promote hope for the future. Particularly related to crises, reframing can be used to assist clients in changing their perception of a situation from one of threat to one of challenge; from one of hopelessness to one of hope; and from something negative to something positive.

3. *Promote perceived control.* Human development is dependent on individuals perceiving that they have some control over their lives. Although nurses may believe that clients have control over what happens to them, many clients do not perceive that they have any control. The nurse must make every effort to promote the client's *perception* of control.

4. *Promote strengths.* Identification and promotion of strengths is a means of assisting clients to mobilize their own resources. In the face of stressors, individuals may become overwhelmed with their perceived weaknesses and not be able to identify or utilize strengths.

5. *Set mutual goals that are health directed.* Nurses must utilize the individual's innate drive to be as healthy as that individual can be. The nurse's and client's goals are the same—to meet the client's basic needs. When the nurse's and client's goals appear to differ, the nurse has most likely not fully modeled the client's world.

Self-Care

Clients' self-care is an important component of the theory. There are three aspects to the concept of self-care: self-care knowledge; self-care resources; and self-care action.

Self-Care Knowledge In most situations, individuals can describe what they perceive as their health problem; they can also identify what they think will make them feel better. In an analysis of case studies reported by Erickson (1990), four themes were found to relate to the nature of self-care knowledge:

1. An individual's perceptions of factors associated with her personal health problems are rarely obvious to the health care provider

2. The individual's perceptions of what is needed to help him can best be defined by that person

3. A nurse's role is to facilitate clients to articulate what they perceive to be associated with their problem and what can be done to help them feel better

4. Another nurse's role is to assist the clients to resolve their problems in ways that meet personal needs and are health- and growth-directed (Erickson, 1990).

Self-Care Resources   All individuals have internal and external resources (strengths and support) that will help gain, maintain, and promote an optimum level of holistic health. It is important for the nurse to assess these resources to assist the client in self-care action.

Self-Care Action   Self-care action is the development and utilization of self-care knowledge and self-care resources. The basis of nursing is assisting clients in self-care action in relation to health.

Affiliated-Individuation

Within the Modeling and Role-Modeling theory, all individuals are seen as having simultaneous needs to be attached to other individuals and to be separate from them. This concept is described in Modeling and Role-Modeling as affiliated-individuation and is considered to be a motivation for human behavior. Affiliated-individuation occurs when "a person perceives himself or herself as simultaneously close to and separate from a significant other" (Erickson et al., 1983, p. 68).

Adaptive Potential

Adaptive potential refers to the individual's ability to mobilize resources to cope with stressors. The Adaptive Potential Assessment Model (APAM) has three categories: equilibrium,

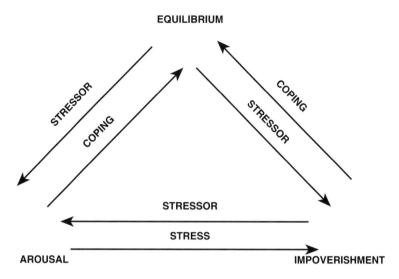

An illustration of the dynamic relationship among the states of the adaptive potential assessment model

---

FIGURE 1.2 The adaptive potential model.

From Erickson, H., Tomlin, E., and Swain, M.A. (1983). *Modeling and Role-Modeling: A theory and paradigm for nursing.* Lexington, SC: Pine Press of Lexington, Inc. Used with permission.

arousal, and impoverishment. Equilibrium has two possibilities: adaptive equilibrium and maladaptive equilibrium. Adaptive potential is dynamic; individuals can move from any of the three states to any of the other states (see figure 1.2). Movement among the states is influenced by the individual's ability to cope.

The APAM identifies states (not traits) of coping, which can assist the nurse in planning interventions for the client. Assessment of adaptive potential has been well-documented (Erickson & Swain, 1982; Barnfather, Swain, & Erickson, 1989; Campbell, Finch, Erickson, & Swain, 1985). Interventions can be guided by the individual's ability to mobilize his own resources.

A person who is impoverished is not in a situation to be an autonomous, independent person eager to learn and to perform self-care. An impoverished person requires affiliation needs to be met, internal strengths to be promoted, and external resources to be provided. A client in arousal is in a stress state and has difficulty mobilizing resources. This client has stronger individuation needs and responds to guidance, direction, assistance, and teaching aimed at self-care.

The client in equilibrium is in a nonstress state. Adaptive equilibrium is different from maladaptive equilibrium in that the adaptive client has all subsystems in harmony, while the maladaptive client is placing one or more subsystems in jeopardy to maintain equilibrium. The importance of equilibrium, whether adaptive or maladaptive, is that the client sees no reason to change since equilibrium exists. Interventions for the client in maladaptive equilibrium need to focus on motivation strategies to develop a desire for change. The APAM model is quite useful in understanding the client in crisis situation. The nurse will first assess for arousal or equilibrium; interventions can then be planned accordingly.

Goals of Nursing Interventions

In dealing with clients in crisis situations, it is imperative to promote the client's control. A crisis often leaves the client with a sense of powerlessness and feelings of anxiety that coincide with experiencing the unpredictable and the unknown.

Whether the crisis is a result of an acute situation (such as a physical injury) or a long-term emotional one (such as grieving the loss of a loved one), nursing interventions have two goals: to increase the client's sense of worth and perception of control, and to promote resolution that will promote a sense of peace and well-being. The Modeling and Role-Modeling theory provides an excellent framework from which to achieve these goals.

SUMMARY

In this chapter, we propose a new look at crisis intervention. The nurse as healer seeks to understand the crisis event in terms of its impact on the whole client, and will use this understanding to assist the client to turn crisis into a growth-producing challenge. The whole client is viewed as both a person having physical, emotional, mental, and spiritual components, and as an integrated whole. The Modeling and Role-Modeling theory is used as the framework to understand the client holistically and to guide nursing practice.

A crisis is an individual, subjective experience. Not all individuals will perceive the same circumstance to be a crisis, and crises can be short-term, acute situations or chronic conditions. The ultimate goal of nursing interventions is to promote optimum health. The American Holistic Nurses Association (AHNA) defines health as a harmony and balance between the physical, emotional, and spiritual components of the individual. From such a holistic perspective, health can be seen in terms of well-being and balance. The nurse, then, understands that although the experience of coping with a crisis is unpleasant, resolution of the crisis may produce great benefits for the individual. On this basis, the authors propose that all crises can and should be viewed in terms of challenges.

References

American Holistic Nurses Association. (1992). *Description of holistic nursing.* Raleigh, NC: Author.

Baird, S.F. (1976). Crisis intervention theory in maternal-infant nursing. *JOGN Nursing, 5*(1), 37–39.

Barnfather, J.S., Swain, M.A.P., & Erickson, H.C. (1989). Construct validity of an aspect of the coping process: Potential adaptation to stress. *Issues in Mental Health Nursing, 10,* 23–40.

Barnfather, J.S., Swain, M.A.P., & Erickson, H.C. (1989). Evaluation of two assessment techniques for adaptation to stress. *Nursing Science Quarterly, 2*(4), 172–182.

Berger, K.J., & Williams, M.B. (1992). *Fundamentals of nursing.* Norwalk, CT: Appleton & Lange.

Campbell, J., Finch, D., Erickson, H., & Swain, M.A.P. (1985). A theoretical approach to nursing assessment. *Journal of Advanced Nursing, 10,* 111–115.

Cross, J.R. (1990). Betty Newman. In J. George (Ed.), *Nursing theories* (pp. 259–278). Norwalk, CT: Appleton & Lange.

Cunningham, J.M. (1991). Crisis intervention. In G. McFarland & M.D. Thomas (Eds.), *Psychiatric mental health nursing* (pp. 759–765). Philadelphia: J.B. Lippincott.

Erickson, H. (1990). Self-care knowledge: An exploratory study. *Modeling and Role-Modeling: Theory, research and practice, 1*(1), 178–202. (Monograph published by the Society for the Advancement of Modeling and Role Modeling.)

Erickson, H., & Swain, M.A. (1982). A model for assessing potential adaptation to stress. *Research in Nursing and Health, 5*, 93–101.

Erickson, H., Tomlin, E., & Swain, M.A. (1983). *Modeling and Role-Modeling: A theory and paradigm for nursing.* Lexington, SC: Pine Press.

Falco, S.M., & Lobo, M.L. (1990). Martha E. Rogers. In J. George (Ed.), *Nursing theories* (pp. 211–230). Norwalk, CT: Appleton & Lange.

Frisch, N., & Bowman, S. (1995). The Modeling and Role-Modeling theory. In J. George (Ed.), *Nursing theories* (4th ed., pp. 355–371). Norwalk, CT: Appleton & Lange.

Fryback, P.B. (1993). Health for people with a terminal diagnosis. *Nursing Science Quarterly, 6*(3), 147–159.

Oxford English Dictionary. (1971). Oxford, England: Oxford University Press.

Stuart, G.W., & Sundeen, S.J. (1991). *Principles and practice of psychiatric nursing.* St. Louis: Mosby Year Book.

Webster's New World Dictionary (2nd college ed.). (1982). New York: Simon and Schuster.

THE
BODY-MIND-
SPIRIT

2

PHYSICAL
CHALLENGES
TO HEALTH

Health care is most frequently provided to clients experiencing physical disease. Any physical ailment perceived to be significant by a person demands reaction and response. One cannot ignore a body that is hurting or exhibiting symptoms. When special challenges must be faced, extra dedication needed to perform tasks, or greater effort exerted to get through the day, then the physical ailment produces a crisis for the person.

What level of physical illness will produce a crisis, and which of the three holistic components—body, mind, or spirit—will be most acutely affected by the crisis will vary among clients. Although the holistic model presented in chapter 1 emphasizes the interconnectedness of body, mind, and spirit, for purposes of exploring how persons cope with challenges, it is helpful to identify the initial event as primarily a crisis of one component of the whole person so that interventions can be tailored accordingly.

Challenges to the physical body include acute and chronic illness, as well as accidental injury. These are inevitable challenges of life. Despite our society's emphasis on health promotion, at some point persons can expect to become ill. The difficulty faced by the average person is that when these physical ailments are encountered, no one ever seems to expect them—they become part of life's surprises. While illness and injury are quite distinct events, there are some common themes present in situations of physical ailments. Life patterns are interrupted and change is demanded. The greater the interruption, the longer the interruption exists. The more demanding the situation, the more likely it will be for the person to see herself in crisis, or as needing nursing support. During this time of physical crisis, a person cannot take bodily health or functioning for granted and becomes conscious of the body's health status. A person may take on the *sick role*, concluding that there is a condition for which treatment is necessary. Willingness to take on that role, however, may vary greatly among people. Internal conflicts over seeing oneself as *ill* or in the sick role may in and of itself produce a crisis for some.

Increasingly, individuals are beginning to see physical challenges as times for reflection and change. Illness requires one to step out of one's day-to-day pattern, to take time out to assess one's life, one's activities. For nurses to support clients undergoing such experiences, particularly for nurses utilizing the Modeling and Role-Modeling theory, it is important that nurses understand the experience from the clients' perspective. There is an emerging body of nursing literature examining clients' experiences of illness. As nurses explore that literature, they gain depth in understanding the subjective, human experiences of clients with whom they work.

THE EXPERIENCE OF ILLNESS

Nurses have a desire and need to understand the rich experiences of their clients' lives. As part of their heritage, nurses have listened to clients tell of personal, human reactions to illness, injury, hospitalization, and treatment. The nurse at the bedside or in the home is in a position to offer care and support consistent with each individual's experiences and views. As nurses seek out and document clients' stories, they have become aware of the impact that subjective experience has on the progress and outcome of the illness or recovery and the need for further understanding of this experience-illness relationship.

Nurses have two sources available for increasing their understanding of how clients experience illness. First, nurses as human beings share the same array of life experiences as their clients and can learn by examining their own experiences of physical illness or injury. Self-understanding is the first requirement for true understanding of others. Second, qualitative research studies are being undertaken whereby one documents the full, lived subjective experiences that clients have regarding their physical health.

The following exercise is presented to help the holistic nurse evaluate her own responses to physical illness or limitations. Acknowledging her own responses helps the nurse to separate her experiences and expectations from those of the client. This enables her to be truly open, not only listening to the client's story but hearing the client's interpretation of the story.

EXERCISE

Examination of One's Subjective Experience of Illness

Consider a time in your life where you became ill or injured to the point where your life patterns were disrupted and you had to make a change in day-to-day living. Remember your experiences, and consider the following questions:

1. Who was the first person you told that you thought you were ill?

2. Did you hesitate in disclosing yourself as ill to others?

3. What led up to you consulting a physician or health care provider?

4. How did you adapt to the role of patient?

- Did you want to direct your care?
- Did you want others to care for you?
- Did you tell them?

5. When did you tell your boss/professional colleagues that you could not carry out your responsibilities; i.e., that you had to stay home, go to the hospital, or take time out for a medical or surgical procedure?

- What were your emotions in talking to your boss?

6. When you remained separated from work and/or social activities because of illness or injury, what were your feelings?

7. Did you examine your life patterns and priorities when you were ill?

PHASES OF THE ILLNESS EXPERIENCE

From the literature on clients' experiences of illness, several themes emerge in nurses' attempts to understand illness. Charmaz (1973) described persons with chronic illness as moving through three phases of experience of the illness. These phases are illness as an interruption, an intrusion, and an encapsulating event. We will suggest that these categories provide a framework for the nurse to observe and interpret all illness.

Illness can be viewed as an interruption in the person's life. In this regard, illness is an unwanted, unexpected occurrence that stops or alters the flow of one's day-to-day life. If the illness is an acute, short-term condition, the interruption may be negligible, creating some anxiety and adjustment but avoiding major adjustments of crisis proportions. However, even short-term, nonserious illness can create a crisis in a person's life if the illness comes at a time of a significant personal event. Consider the times we have all heard someone say, "I just can't handle having the flu today!" "There couldn't be a worse time for me to have a cold than now." "But I can't be sick, I have the most important meetings of the year scheduled tomorrow." Clearly, the severity of the illness does not dictate the client's response to it. The nurse must consider the illness within the context of the client's life, learning by listening to what the client's perception is of the interruption caused by the condition.

Secondly, illness can move from being an interruption to being an intrusion. As an intrusion, the physical condition becomes an imposition, an encroachment on the person's life. Typically, an illness becomes intrusive when it doesn't go away, when the condition is long-term or chronic. Persons experiencing illness as intrusive describe the physical condition as the focus of their thoughts and activities. They have less time and/or energy for other endeavors; they wish for involvement, but are inhibited because of their limitations.

Lastly, particularly for chronic illness, the physical condition moves into a phase where the person feels encapsulated by the illness. Here, the person feels caught or entrapped because the physical condition has taken over his life. Major adjustments to living are required as daily routines are formed to adapt to the treatment. The person is challenged to break out into a new equilibrium in order to reach a new balance. The client will have new boundaries, all dictated by the illness. Needless to say, a condition that causes feelings of encapsulation will affect every person close to the client as well. Table 2.1 summarizes the concepts of illness/physical limitation as interruption, intrusion, and encapsulating event with criteria for nursing assessments.

STUDIES OF THE EXPERIENCE OF ILLNESS

Other information about persons' experiences of illness come from an array of studies, each of which has tried to document the experience of a particular client group. A phenomenological study that set out to provide a portrait of what it is like to be ill revealed that clients experience illness as alienating, creating uncertainty and feelings of despair (Kretlow, 1990). A qualitative study of women diagnosed with breast cancer suggested that illness demands are felt in every aspect of a woman's life, including her identity, daily

Perception of Illness	Symptoms	Responses
Interruption	Flow of life is stopped. Life patterns are blocked.	Surprise; Anger; Annoyance
Intrusion	Physical condition is the focus of activities. Immediate life goals are blocked.	Anxiety; Isolation
Encapsulating event	Physical condition is the only focus of thoughts for days or weeks.	Fear; Powerlessness; Obsessions r/t physical state

TABLE 2.1 Perceptions of Illness, Client Symptoms, and Responses

routines, family and social experiences, and her perception of the past, present, and future (Loveys & Klaich, 1991). A similar study of adults with chronic respiratory illnesses found that clients experiencing dyspnea experience fear, helplessness, loss of vitality, preoccupation, and legitimacy (DeVito, 1990).

In a qualitative study of pregnant women requiring bedrest, Maloni et al. (1993) found that the separation from family was the client's most important concern. Further, women in the study expressed concerns about health, their body image, their family status, and emotional changes.

In an investigation of persons with chronic illness, Pollack (1993) found that illnesses that were more likely to involve physical disabilities (such as multiple sclerosis) were perceived to be more of a burden than those that did not (such as hypertension). Further, Pollack reported that adaptation to the physical illness was easier for conditions that are constant as opposed to those that are progressive or unpredictable.

In another study, Fryback (1993) evaluated clients with terminal illnesses and found that the experience of a life-threatening illness served as a catalyst for these individuals to make significant changes in their lives. These individuals learned to view health holistically, and defined themselves as healthy, despite the fact that they had a physical ailment.

It becomes clear that physical illness is an uncomfortable experience accompanied by strong emotions such as isolation, fear, alienation, uncertainty, and helplessness. There are times when significant illness serves as a catalyst for positive growth (Fryback, 1993) and times when the positive growth does not or cannot occur. While there are many individual factors associated with why this positive outcome may or may not result, it is important to look at what is known about how persons successfully adapt to physical illness.

In the case of chronic illness, Miller (1992) lists 13 coping tasks that clients must address to successfully integrate the illness into their lives and functioning. These tasks are:

1. Maintaining a sense of normalcy
2. Modifying daily routine, adjusting lifestyle
3. Obtaining knowledge and skill for continuing self-care
4. Maintaining a positive concept of self

5. Adjusting to altered social relationships
6. Grieving over losses concomitant with chronic illness
7. Dealing with role change
8. Handling physical discomfort
9. Complying with prescribed regimen
10. Confronting the inevitability of one's own death
11. Dealing with social stigma of illness or disability
12. Maintaining a feeling of being in control
13. Maintaining hope despite uncertain or downward course of health. (p. 27)

These tasks provide a series of challenges clients must meet. The role of the nurse helping a client with physical illness must be to strive to understand the client's perception of the illness, to understand the illness from within the context of the client's life, and to plan interventions that support the client's coping and positive adjustment to meet these challenges.

USING THE MODELING AND ROLE-MODELING THEORY TO PLAN CARE

The Modeling and Role-Modeling theory helps the nurse to direct care that is supportive and nurturing for the client (Erickson, Tomlin, & Swain, 1983). The nurse begins by meeting the client and focusing on the client's needs, worries, and wants. The nurse must remember that at some level clients know what made them ill, and they also know what is needed to make them well.

Starting with the five aims of intervention (see chapter 1), the nurse must build trust and initiate a positive nurse-client relationship. The nurturing role of the nurse emphasizes acceptance of the client and a readiness to meet the client's needs. In situations of physical illness, the nurse begins by providing immediate, physical care, asking the client what is wanted or needed, and listening to the client's concerns and perceptions. The nurse understands that illness will be perceived differently by each person, and that the level of interruption, intrusion, and sense of encapsulation felt may have much more to do with the client's life patterns, beliefs, and values than with the medical diagnosis.

The Adaptive Potential Model, a concept within the Modeling and Role-Modeling theory, can serve as a valuable framework for evaluating the client's adaptive state of equilibrium, arousal, or impoverishment. In figure 2.1, Bowman (1992) summarizes this process, demonstrating how the nurse may analyze information to

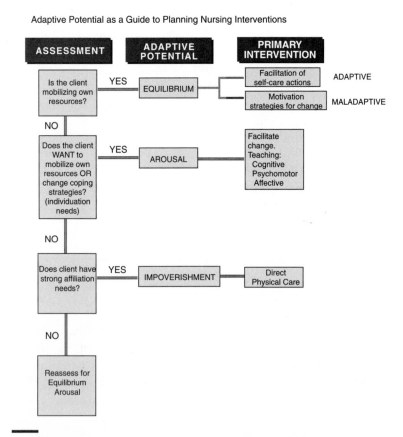

Adaptive Potential as a Guide to Planning Nursing Interventions

FIGURE 2.1 *Adaptive potential as a guide to planning nursing interventions.*

Presented at the Fourth International Modeling and Role-Modeling Conference, 1992. (Susan S. Bowman, Humboldt State University. Used with permission.)

conclude the client's state of adaptive potential. If the client is in adaptive equilibrium, nursing actions are supportive; if the client is in maladaptive equilibrium, nursing actions are to motivate for change. If the client is in arousal, nursing actions are to facilitate change by assisting the client to mobilize his own resources to cope. If the client is in a state of impoverishment, the nurse should begin by providing direct physical care and help the client to identify perceived resources.

The Modeling and Role-Modeling theory provides a framework for the nurse to better understand nursing from a new perspective. If a client is experiencing illness as a crisis, the client will be in arousal or in impoverishment. For many nurses, it is easier to identify a crisis state in a client experiencing arousal than in the client in impoverishment. The client in arousal will demonstrate anxiety and be engaged in coping activities; the client in impoverishment will appear passive. One must not interpret impoverishment as the *quiet and compliant client,* for the client in impoverishment is exhausted of resources and needs considerable nursing care to begin to adapt to his current situation.

Once the level of adaptive potential is known, the nurse can assess the client's coping methods, and help the client to evaluate which means of coping are most effective. Use of the theory requires that the nurse understand the world from the client's perspective, that is, the nurse makes a model of the client's world. This is modeling—entering into another's perspective, seeing and interpreting the illness and the surrounding events as the client sees them. Next, the nurse must role-model healthy coping behaviors that will draw on the client's own resources and move the client toward adaptive equilibrium. (The case study in this chapter provides illustrations of these concepts.)

NURSING DIAGNOSIS

Nurses express the nursing concerns in diagnostic language so that a standard care plan can be made. Dealing with physical illness, the physiological diagnoses will be readily established. The diagnoses that need to be uncovered are those assessing

the client's emotional responses to the physical illness—
those concerns such as fear or anxiety, social isolation, and
impaired body image—which indicate that the experience of
physical illness evokes significant human responses on an
emotional level that must be addressed before the physical body
can or will heal.

CASE STUDY | *Fred*

(Adapted from Wendy Woodward, Humboldt State
University, personal communication, 1993. Used with permission.)

Fred is a 68-year-old white male, a retired engineer
who was admitted to the hospital for a right carotid
endarterectomy. His medical history includes: CAD,
severe; MI at age 43 years (he was told at age 43 years
that he had the circulatory system of an 80 year old);
has had two small strokes, leaving him with foot drop
in left foot and one calf muscle smaller than the other.
He has a personal history of both drinking and smoking, although he quit drinking five years ago and
smoking four years ago. He takes antihypertensive
medications and aspirin daily. He lives with his wife.
They have three grown children who live on their own
in locations throughout the state in which Fred lives.
His lifestyle is sedentary; he used to read extensively
but no longer reads much. He is 5'11" tall, weighs 135
pounds, B.P. 140/96, H/H and all other lab reports are
within normal limits.

The morning of the scheduled surgery, Fred's
BUN and creatinine were elevated. Consultation with

his physician regarding the lab work delayed his surgery six hours. Fred's anxiety about the surgical procedure increased during the delay. He expressed ambivalence about the procedure, but gave consent for the operation.

On the operating table, his BP rose to 280/140 and he had a massive, left-sided stroke. He was placed on a respirator for impaired breathing patterns. Nurses received him in ICU and identified his priorities as: maintaining airway, monitoring BP, urine output, LOC, and assessing for pain and fear. They proceeded to provide care as appropriate for these priorities. Fred progressed physically and within 3 weeks was placed in a stepdown unit and rehabilitation planning was initiated. Fred had had a left-sided stroke, leaving his right side impaired. He could stand only with assistance, he could not use his dominant hand, his visual field was diminished, and he had a right-sided sensory deficit. The nurses carrying out interventions for Fred's rehabilitation noted that he was angry and hostile, he was "overly concerned" with his urine output, and he wanted to urinate frequently. He was easily frustrated and did not communicate well with anyone at the hospital. His wife was at the end of her rope, and she expressed feeling guilty that he was such a difficult client. At this point, Fred's nursing care plan was developed and was aimed at keeping him active and involved. The initial nursing care plan is presented in table 2.2. Nurses were consistent in carrying out the interventions. Fred did not improve; he only became more upset and hostile.

At this point, holistic nurse Myra entered the case and evaluated Fred from the point of view of Modeling and Role-Modeling, understanding that the physical

Nursing Diagnosis	Goal	Interventions
Activity intolerance r/t illness and debilitated state	Accomplish ADLs Controlled mobility	Gradual increase of activity; ambulate QID; utilization of aids (walker)
Social isolation r/t lack of contact with others	Return to premorbid. level of socialization	Ward placement; therapy: personal/group; reinforce social contact with family, especially wife
Sensory deficit r/t paralysis and visual field alteration	Positive adaptation to sensory losses	Training with ADLs; compensation with lipped plates, turning food tray; adaptive equipment; feed as needed
Altered elimination r/t atonic bladder	Patient will not be incontinent of urine	Offer urinal q 1 hour; assess for UTI
Nutrition: less than body requirements	Adequate nutrition Stable body weight	Offer supplements

TABLE 2.2   Initial Nursing Care Plan for Fred

illness might well be a crisis for Fred and that his care needed to be individualized based on his worldview.

The first consideration for Myra was the meaning of the experiences of illness, surgery, and the stroke to Fred. The second consideration was what Fred wanted in terms of recovery. Myra began by approaching Fred with an attitude of unconditional acceptance, willing to provide nurturance in whatever form Fred found acceptable. These actions are consistent with the five aims of intervention, starting from a place of building trust. Myra assessed Fred's adaptive potential, and concluded that he was in arousal. He was frustrated and angry, with an escalating anxiety level. He was showing his state of arousal by being hostile and uncooperative. On one level, Fred was appealing to the nurses to notice him, to listen to him.

Myra assessed that the experience of illness was a crisis for Fred at this time. The experience of this illness was an encapsulating event. He was obsessed with urination in response to feeling completely out of control. Fred was responding to the crisis in the only way he could. His method of coping was to attempt to mobilize his resources. However, because of his debilitated state, the nursing staff were resources he had to use to accomplish anything. He wanted to direct his care, to feel independent, but he was not given the chance to do that. He wanted the nurses to know that he did not wish to be subjected to group therapy and social activities, nor did he wish to have his day so solidly structured with rehabilitation activities.

What did he want? Myra had to talk with him, spending time learning of his worries, needs, and wants. In time, he communicated with her, as he recognized that she wanted to help him begin to direct his own care. Fred had been an engineer; he was used to being in control of events. He liked having information to assist him in making his own decisions. He wanted someone to understand that he was tired, that his condition made him feel helpless, that he was experiencing the loss of his independence and his control over his life, and that he no longer liked his body.

Myra completely revised his nursing care plan. While not ignoring Fred's physiological needs, his needs for safety, nutrition, and elimination, the new and revised nursing diagnoses focused on Fred's subjective concerns. The priority diagnoses became fatigue, powerlessness, body-image disturbance, and grieving. Table 2.3 presents Myra's care plan. With this new approach, all nursing care was directed to Fred's feelings, and the care helped Fred to regain control. With the new approach, Fred was permitted to explore his own feelings, to identify his resources, and to begin to direct his own rehabilitation.

Nursing Diagnosis	Goal	Interventions
Fatigue r/t illness, and debilitated state	Provide balance btw rest, sleep, and activities	Permit Fred to set his own pace, allow him to set his daily schedule. Give uninterrupted time to sit quietly. Offer interventions to elicit the relaxation response (massage, guided relaxation, TT, healing touch).
Powerlessness r/t loss of control over his life's events	Increase Fred's perception of control	Allow Fred to set daily schedule. Provide Fred with control over daily events.
Body-image disturbance r/t paralysis and debilitated state	Fred will accept his physical condition	Emphasize strengths. Permit honest discussion of feelings.
Grieving r/t losses (health, mobility, independence, youth)	Fred will accept the loss of health and embark on a path toward rehabilitation	Encourage Fred to describe the loss of health, youth, independence. Share grief with him.

TABLE 2.3   *Revised Nursing Care Plan for Fred*

Fred was put in control, and the nurses became resources he could use.

Discussion

One important principle of crisis intervention is that the nurse should allow the client to have a sense of control. The difficulty in the case of Fred was that the nurses did not readily view the physical illness as a crisis, so they did not identify Fred as being in a crisis state. Nurses assumed Fred was ready to embark on a rehabilitative plan for recovery. A person in crisis is unable to do this. Once the crisis was identified by Myra, nursing actions and an alternative nursing approach became clear. This example provides an illustration of how the Modeling and Role-Modeling theory and the concept of physical illness as a crisis can provide a framework for nursing assessment and planning. Care under this model becomes holistic, client-centered, and compassionate—a goal of all nursing.

SUMMARY

Physical illnesses challenge the health and peace of our clients. Charmaz (1973) suggested that illness (or crisis in general) is subjectively experienced in one of three phases: interruption, intrusion, or encapsulation. These phases are based on the level of encroachment on the client's life. Studies document the client's experience of illness as a basis to understanding the varied meanings of physical illness to individuals. Using the Modeling and Role-Modeling theory, the holistic nurse can understand the client's challenges and assist him in regaining balance and health.

References

Bowman, S. (1992, October). *Adaptive potential as a guide to planning nursing interventions.* Presented at the Fourth National Modeling and Role-Modeling Conference, Boston, MA.

Charmaz, K. (1973). *Time and identity: The shaping of selves of the chronically ill.* Unpublished doctoral dissertation. University of California, San Francisco, CA.

DeVito, A.J. (1990). Dyspnea during hospitalization for acute phase of illness as recalled by patients with chronic, obstructive pulmonary disease. *Heart and Lung, 19*(2), 186–191.

Erickson, H., Tomlin, E., & Swain, M.A. (1983). *Modeling and Role-Modeling: A theory and paradigm for nursing.* Lexington, SC: Pine Press.

Fryback, P.B. (1993). Health for people with a terminal illness. *Nursing Science Quarterly, 6*(3), 147–159.

Kretlow, F. (1990). A phenomenological view of illness. *Australian Journal of Advanced Nursing, 7*(2), 8–10.

Loveys, B.J., & Klaich, K. (1991). Breast cancer: Demands of illness. *Oncology Nurses Forum, 18*(1), 75–80.

Maloni, J., Chance, B., Zhang, C., Cohen, A.W., Betts, D., & Gange, S.T. (1993). Physical and psychosocial side effects of antepartum hospital bed rest. *Nursing Research, 42*(4), 197–203.

Miller, J.F. (1992). *Coping with chronic illness, overcoming powerlessness* (2nd ed.). Philadelphia: F.A. Davis.

Pollack, S.E. (1993). Adaptation to chronic illness: A program of research for testing nursing theory. *Nursing Science Quarterly, 6*(2), 86–92.

3 MENTAL AND EMOTIONAL CHALLENGES TO HEALTH

Can mental images and an individual's sense of choice promote health and peace? Many today would answer "yes," particularly in situations where one's emotional and mental responses to stimuli result in an inward sense of balance and harmony. The converse is also true—that mental images and emotional reactions can interfere with peace, and in some instances result in physical or psychological illness.

CHALLENGES POSING EMOTIONAL OR MENTAL THREATS

Mental anguish is displayed differently by different persons, but it is a universal human experience. Every one of us has felt the tensions associated with anticipating some important event, the fear of a major decision working against us, the guilt we carry around for being less than perfect, or the sleepless nights we experience when we dwell with worry on unpleasant things that probably won't come to pass. Further, when we are faced with one of life's real challenges—chronic illness, family disputes, unemployment, violence, or unjust acts—our mental responses to the event will work to either help us regain health and peace, or do just the opposite. Table 3.1 presents a list of common situations evoking strong emotional or mental responses. The reader is asked to review the items in the table to find those with which to identify from a personal perspective. Once reviewed, each person can determine which events resonate with one's own experience, and take a few moments to get in touch with the feelings these situations prompted.

For most persons experiencing situations listed in table 3.1, there are strong emotional responses. There are feelings of anger, sadness, fear, disappointment, irritation, and the like. A common theme that underlies these emotions is the sense of a loss of control, the sense of the situation as an unwelcomed intrusion into one's life. In chapter 1, we defined a crisis as a challenge, any event that calls for special effort or dedication. Our emotional and cognitive reactions to these crisis situations will impact significantly on crisis resolution. Let us look, then, at the human reactions to emotional and mental challenges.

EMOTIONAL AND COGNITIVE REACTIONS

Any event that leads to a perceived loss of control compounds the challenge for an individual. There are common human

- Death of a significant other
- Divorce
- Surviving a major accident
- Having a significant physical illness
- Developing a chronic illness
- Losing a job
- Being a victim of violence
- Being a victim of a lawsuit
- Facing a moral/ethical dilemma
- Having to relocate

TABLE 3.1   *Situations Evoking Strong Emotional or Mental Responses*

responses to these situations, and these can be described as nursing diagnoses. These responses are: anxiety or fear, powerlessness, and hopelessness. Examination of these human responses provides insight into the process of going through these experiences.

Nursing Diagnosis: Anxiety/Fear

Anxiety is defined as an unclear or vague feeling whose source is nonspecific or unknown to the individual (North American Nursing Diagnosis Association [NANDA], 1987). Anxiety is accompanied by feelings of tension and/or apprehension. The person experiencing anxiety will describe a sense of impending doom. The physiological response to anxiety includes sympathetic stimulation—cardiovascular excitation, superficial vasoconstriction, and pupil constriction. Behaviors exhibited by the anxious person are restlessness, insomnia, poor eye contact, glancing about, trembling, voice quivering, and facial tension. Fear is distinct from anxiety in that fear is a feeling of dread related to an identifiable source which the person validates. However, the person experiencing fear will exhibit the same responses as one experiencing anxiety.

Persons are thought to experience anxiety whenever there is a threat to one's self-concept, a threat to one's health status, or a crisis situation demanding change in any of life's patterns. Carpenito (1993) identifies that there are cognitive reactions to anxiety. A person may have an inability to concentrate, a lack of awareness of surroundings, forgetfulness or ruminations, orientation to the past, or hyperattentiveness. These cognitive responses are related to the degree of emotional response the individual is experiencing.

There is general agreement that there is a continuum of anxiety responses ranging from mild anxiety to a panic state. These stages of anxiety are described in table 3.2. In mild anxiety, the person experiences the tensions of day-to-day life. He is alert with an increased perceptual field. In moderate anxiety, the person focuses only on immediate concerns, with a narrowed perceptual field. In severe anxiety, the person's perceptual field is greatly reduced and the individual will focus on a specific detail. In a panic state, the person will have feelings of

MILD:	tension of day-to-day living; individual has an alert perceptual field; can motivate learning
MODERATE:	focus is on immediate concerns; perceptual field is narrowed; individual exhibits selective inattention
SEVERE:	focus is on specific detail, and nothing else; perceptual field is greatly reduced
PANIC:	individual experiences a sense of awe, dread, and/or terror; individual loses control; there is disorganization of the personality

TABLE 3.2   Stages of Anxiety

dread or terror, and will be unable to control behaviors. "Panic is a frightening and paralyzing experience" (Stuart & Sundeen, 1991, p. 320).

When working with clients experiencing severe levels of anxiety or fear, the nurse must first be concerned with safety. Providing a calming and secure environment will help relieve some of the client's feelings of dread or terror. Next, the nurse will take measures to support the client's feelings, and permit him to express concerns, move at his own pace, and share feelings or concerns to whatever degree he desires.

Individuals can learn to identify their own anxiety, and discover the events that precipitate anxious responses. In this way, the client can use cognitive skills to balance the affective, emotional states of anxiety and fear.

Nursing Diagnosis: Powerlessness

Powerlessness is a perception that one's own actions will not significantly affect an outcome; a perceived lack of control over a current situation or immediate happening (NANDA, 1987). Persons experiencing powerlessness will express dissatisfaction with their ability to take control and manage events. Persons experiencing powerlessness may exhibit passivity, lack of initiative, and decreased verbalizations.

Situations where persons feel powerless include facing significant illness, inability to perform usual daily tasks, and conditions of obesity or disfigurement. Further, situations where the person is not consulted regarding decisions that affect him, and maturational crises lead to powerlessness as well (Carpenito, 1993).

When providing care, nurses must recognize that power-lessness is a subjective feeling. Hence, in identical situations, one person may see choices where another does not. Nurses must accept the client's feelings as valid, and work with the client to consider options. A person's sense of powerlessness is related to the person's locus of control. Persons with an internal locus of control are able and desire to make their own decisions. They are used to managing themselves, and will be upset if choices are nonexistent. Conversely, persons with an external locus of control are used to having others involved in making decisions for them. Such persons will decide what to do based on others' opinions and expectations. In some situations, a person with an external locus of control will not feel powerless, but a person with an internal locus of control will feel powerless.

Generally, a person with an internal locus of control is more mature, more able to handle life's stressors than one with an external locus of control. However, the role of nursing interventions is to identify the feelings of powerlessness in any individual, determine the situation(s) or event(s) that precipitated the feelings, and assist the client to regain control over his or her own life. Failure to address powerlessness over time leads to feelings of alienation and estrangement.

As in the case of anxiety and fear, persons can choose to view a situation as one with or without choices. Individuals can use their cognitive functioning to open up new ideas and new paths, and to regain a sense of involvement with the environment. Nursing interventions are directed toward this goal.

Nursing Diagnosis: Hopelessness

Hopelessness is defined as a state in which an individual sees limited or no alternatives or personal choices available and is unable to mobilize energy on his own behalf (NANDA, 1987). A person feeling hopeless will demonstrate passivity, decreased verbalization, and decreased affect. Hopelessness differs from power-lessness in that a hopeless person sees no solution to his problem, whereas a powerless person may see an alternative or answer to the problems, but be unable to do anything about it (Carpenito, 1991).

To experience hopelessness is to experience despair, helplessness, sadness, and/or depression. Hope is a quality that sustains life. It is a cognitive behavior that allows one to act; for example, to see a crisis as an opportunity for growth and change. Hope gives a person a sense of future, and belief that a bad situation can improve. "Hope helps a person to feel whole" (Carpenito, 1989, p. 436).

Nursing interventions for a client experiencing hopelessness begin with a compassionate recognition of the client's feelings and subjective experiences. The nurse should evaluate the degree of hopelessness and assess the client's suicide potential. Then, over time from within the grounding of a nurse-patient relationship, the nurse can assist the client to reframe her situation in positive terms. Assisting the client to make choices and decisions promotes a sense of control that the client no longer sees (Ekland, 1991).

DEALING WITH EMOTIONAL AND MENTAL RESPONSES

There are several nursing approaches for intervening with the human mental and emotional responses to challenges and crises. These techniques include relaxation-focused modalities, which aim to promote physiological changes and relieve tension, and cognitive-focused modalities, which aim to replace negative thoughts and perceptions with positive ones. These will be discussed separately.

Relaxation-Focused Modalities

Relaxation is defined as a psychophysiological state characterized by parasympathetic dominance involving multiple visceral and somatic symptoms; the absence of physical, mental, and emotional tension (Dossey, Keegan, Guzzetta, & Kolkmeier, 1988). Relaxation permits a person to quiet himself, retreat mentally from his surroundings, and decrease tension, anxiety, and/or pain. Relaxation is desirable for clients who are undergoing crises or challenges, and for those persons who report feeling tense, irritable, fearful, and/or angry because it allows the person to leave the reality of the threatening event for a short time, and return often with a more objective (therefore, less emotional) view of the world around. While there are many techniques of relaxation, a few of the modalities used regularly by nurses are described.

Progressive Muscle Relaxation (PMR) PMR is a technique of alternately tensing and relaxing muscle groups throughout the body to become aware of tensions and the contrast between muscle tension and relaxation. Persons undergoing PMR are led through sessions by a coach who assists them to a comfortable position and suggests the process of tensing and releasing major muscle groups (working from feet to head). Persons receiving PMR as a treatment are able to get in touch with tensions and become aware of the degree to which these tensions are affecting their physical bodies. Over time, many persons can use PMR as a self-care intervention or with the help of an audiotape.

Imagery Imagery is defined as those "internal experiences of memories, dreams, fantasies, and visions; imagery may involve one, several, or all of the senses and serves as a bridge for connecting body, mind, and spirit" (Dossey et al., 1988, p. 224). Dossey and colleagues further state that imagery is a normal process that evokes change at the cellular level (p. 224). Imagery is often practiced by having the nurse or coach suggest pleasant visualizations to the client to help the client achieve relaxation. For example, a visualization might be to imagine a "special place" where the client feels safe and warm, or to picture oneself on a comfortable beach, or in one's own home where everything is quiet and just the way it should be. In practice, PMR and imagery are often used together, where PMR initiates a relaxation response, and imagery permits the client to use the mind to leave the uncomfortable reality for a more pleasant internal environment.

Nurses have investigated both PMR and imagery in several areas of practice. Holden-Lund (1988) reported on the effects of relaxation and guided imagery (RGI) on the psychophysiologic stress response and wound healing of postcholecystectomy patients. In a controlled study, subjects who participated in RGI had a significantly lowered state of anxiety, lowered cortisol levels, and less superficial wound erythema than controls who had no intervention.

Use of both of these techniques has been widely reported in cancer patients. A group of researchers documented the thought and image patterns of patients undergoing chemotherapy and suggested that a person's emotional reaction to a stressful situation is influenced by that person's perception (Manson, Manderino, & Johnson, 1993). Rancour (1991) reported that guided imagery can be used to bring a sense of healing to a terminal cancer patient. In a review of several research studies utilizing PMR with guided imagery in oncology, Sims (1989) reported that the results are encouraging for practice in helping clients to cope with cancer.

Another group of researchers evaluated PMR and guided imagery for its effect on the psychoimmunological status of bereaved spouses (Houldin, McCorkle, & Lowery, 1993). Results suggested trends in psychoimmunological benefits. Other authors have provided a framework for use of these techniques in other practice situations—Rees for the laboring mother (1992), Dossey, Guzzetta, and Kenner for critical care patients following trauma and surgery (1990). The balance of clinical opinion is that PMR and imagery are valuable, albeit underutilized, nursing interventions. Benefits of the technique include lowering anxiety, easing muscle tension, pain, and fatigue, and assisting clients to sleep (Dossey et al., 1988).

Hypnosis   Hypnosis is a specialized technique that can have a powerful impact on a person's ability to relax. Hypnosis involves inducing an altered state of consciousness for the purpose of changing perception, memory, or sensations (Dossey et al., 1988, p. 196).

Hypnotherapy has been investigated as a treatment for pain (Petterson, Questad, & Boltwood, 1987; Valente, 1991; Zahourek, 1982), as well as a treatment for anxiety (Valente, 1990; Forbes & Pekala, 1993). Although fewer nurses have requisite training to induce hypnotic states than to practice PMR or guided imagery, hypnosis stands as an appropriate nursing intervention for many of our clients.

Cognitive-Focused Modalities

Helping clients replace negative thoughts with more positive ones is the goal of cognitive-focused modalities. One author provides this explanation for a situation for which cognitive-focused modalities are appropriate: "Depressed persons view situations negatively when more positive interpretations are equally valid" (Zerhusen, Boyle, & Wilson, 1991). Thus, the cognitive approach relies on the person's cognitive abilities to alter not the situation but his perception of it.

Cognitive Therapy   Cognitive therapy permits the nurse to address three major aims—to increase the client's sense of control over his goals and behaviors, to increase the client's self-esteem, and to assist the client in modifying negative expectations (Stuart & Sundeen, 1991). This therapy is conducted by teaching the client to understand the role of cognition in contributing to her feelings of anxiety, powerlessness, and hopelessness. Next, the client is taught to identify images that are self-defeating and/or disruptive. The client is then helped to look at alternative interpretations and alternative behaviors that would produce positive emotions. The client is often helped to accomplish this change of perception through role-plays and rehearsals of positive self-statements.

Nurses have investigated the use of cognitive therapy in diverse settings. The approach was first evaluated as a treatment for depression (Campbell, 1992; Hughes, 1991; Johanson, 1991; Zerhusen et al., 1991). It is currently becoming popular for other psychosocial phenomena as well. In a 1991 study, Reeder evaluated its use for anger management.

Cognitive therapy gives the nurse a tool to help clients find a balance between their emotional state and the situation in which they find themselves. It permits the client to see the world from another perspective and reframe the crisis to a challenge, reframe the challenge from an unwanted intrusion to an event of living.

Attitudinal Healing   Attitudinal healing is an approach developed by Jampolsky to assist persons facing the crisis of a life-threatening illness. The philosophy of attitudinal healing is presented in Jampolsky's popular writings (1979). The idea is based on the belief that it is possible for any person to choose peace rather than conflict, and love rather than fear. Attitudinal healing is the process of letting go of painful and fearful attitudes. Attitudinal healing uses a support group approach, where individuals come together to provide acceptance, love, and support to each other, with the help of a trained volunteer acting as group facilitator. There are twelve Principles of Attitudinal Healing (see table 3.3) that help individuals learn a new, very positive way of thinking about the world in which they find themselves.

Although the approach was first developed for persons with life-threatening illnesses, attitudinal healing groups now work with clients with numerous other concerns. Many persons who have participated in attitudinal healing report that the experience changed their outlook. Indeed, they report that the experience changed the quality of their lives. To date, however, there are no published studies on the effects of attitudinal healing. The closest research that exists indicates that support groups are beneficial to cancer patients (Speigel, Bloom, Kraement, & Gottheil, 1989). The authors' experience is that attitudinal healing is a powerful, positive modality. Nurses are encouraged to investigate this approach for use with clients undergoing challenges and living life's crises.

---

1. The essence of our being is love.
2. Health is inner peace. Healing is letting go of fear.
3. Giving and receiving are the same.
4. We can let go of our past and of the future.
5. Now is the only time there is and each instant is for giving.
6. We can learn to love ourselves and others by forgiving rather than judging.
7. We can become love finders rather than fault finders.
8. We can choose and direct ourselves to be peaceful inside regardless of what is happening outside.
9. We are students and teachers to each other.
10. We can focus on the whole of life rather than on the fragments.
11. Since love is eternal, death need not be viewed as fearful.
12. We can always perceive others as either extending love or giving a call for help.

TABLE 3.3   *Principles of Attitudinal Healing*
Used with permission. The Center for Attitudinal Healing, Sausalito, CA.

NURSING THEORY AND MENTAL/EMOTIONAL RESPONSES

The Modeling and Role-Modeling theory (Erickson, Tomlin, & Swain, 1983) provides a good theoretical base for the nurse who is addressing the nursing diagnoses discussed here, and who is using the interventions described. The theory suggests that the nurse must first understand the client's world and model that world in order to facilitate health behaviors. The goal of the theory is to empower clients to accomplish what they want. The aims of interventions begin with building trust and promoting positive self-regard. A nurse evaluating a client who is experiencing anxiety and fear related to the diagnosis of a life-threatening illness can use this theory to apply the nursing process. The following case study provides an example.

CASE STUDY | *Amy*

Amy is a 40-year-old woman with a medical diagnosis of breast cancer. She is married with two children, ages 12 and 14 years. She has had no previous illnesses and has been active and involved in her community. She works part-time at the city library and participates in a variety of civic groups. There is no history of breast cancer in her family; her diagnosis was made after she noticed a small breast lump, for which she immediately sought medical attention. She underwent mammography and biopsy, followed by lumpectomy surgery. For Amy, the diagnosis of cancer made a significant impact on her view of herself; the diagnosis was a turning point in her life—a point after which everything she did and planned reflected a "new Amy."

Amy was referred to a support group for women with cancer, and she attended readily. She was tearful and emotional during her first meeting with the others. She stated she could not get past the idea of cancer to feel she could go on living the rest of her life normally. She felt she was experiencing shock. She demonstrated both anxiety and fear and readily reached out to the others for support.

Amy was surprised to learn that most of the others in the group had been dealing with a cancer diagnosis for a longer period of time than she had, and that many had a much poorer prognosis than she had. The others told her at her first meeting that the challenge is to live each day fully and not dwell on the diagnoses or the endless lists of "what if . . ." problems.

Using the Modeling and Role-Modeling theory, the nurse who facilitated the group (Maria) assessed that Amy was in a state of arousal. Amy was frightened and felt alone. She was emphasizing the negative connotations of her medical diagnosis and was ruminating on the fact that cancer means a terminal illness. She was also thinking of all the reasons that it was unfair that she (as opposed to all the healthy women in the community) would have a cancerous lump in her breast. She told the other group members, both by her words and her behaviors, that she wanted support. Maria believed that Amy was mobilizing her resources and reaching out to the help provided through the support group.

Maria further assessed that Amy had an internal locus of control and was asking health care providers what she could do to help her condition. Hence, she readily went to the support group. Her anxiety was at a moderate level. Her mental response to her condition was to compound negative thoughts. The nursing care plan included the diagnoses of: anxiety r/t to the unknown long-term outcome of cancer treatment; fear of death and the experience of terminal illness; powerlessness r/t having to confront a significant illness—a situation over which Amy had no choice. Maria believed that the support group would serve as a cognitive therapy, as well as a social and emotional support for Amy. Maria encouraged her to continue attending.

Amy attended the weekly group sessions for two months. By the second meeting, Amy was able to listen to another woman's concerns and offer verbal support— something she was unable to do during the first meeting. By the end of her third group meeting, Amy learned to reframe some of her thinking so she could focus on her day-to-day activities, rather than on her illness. She learned this by hearing and seeing others do the same, and by being willing to give up negative thoughts for positive ones. Slowly, over the next few weeks, Amy was able to focus her attention on the quality of her living—her family life, her work, her friendships. She had periods of feeling angry or feeling depressed that she had breast cancer. When these feelings emerged, she was able to feel the emotion and recognize that others in her situation feel similarly. She was also able to acknowledge that these feelings were acceptable, but she did not have to let these feelings dictate her life. She became a woman who was dealing with an illness, but still living in a world that offered her many positive experiences. Thus, the support group and the cognitive therapy offered helped Amy to resolve, not the physical condition of the cancer, but her mental and emotional reaction to it.

SUMMARY

Mental anguish is a universal human experience, and the emotional discomfort one feels from challenges to the mind is great. In this chapter, we explored the meaning of mental and emotional challenges and examined the common human responses to those challenges. Nursing diagnoses of anxiety, fear, hopelessness, and powerlessness were reviewed to provide insight to the feelings of clients. Interventions specific to the emotional, attitudinal, and cognitive components of a person were addressed. Finally, the case study of a woman undergoing emotional and cognitive reponses to a medical diagnosis of cancer was presented to illustrate a supportive and effective nursing role.

References

Campbell, J.M. (1992). Treating depression in well older adults. *Issues in Mental Health Nursing, 13*(1), 19–29.

Carpenito, L.J. (1989). *Nursing diagnosis: Application to practice.* (3rd ed.). Philadelphia: J.B. Lippincott.

Carpenito, L.J. (1993). *Nursing diagnosis: Application to practice.* (5th ed.). Philadelphia: J.B. Lippincott.

Dossey, B., Guzzetta, C., & Kenner, C. (1990). *Essentials of critical care nursing.* Philadelphia: J.B. Lippincott.

Dossey, B., Keegan, L., Guzzetta, C., & Kolkmeier, L. (1988). *Holistic nursing—A handbook for practice.* Rockville, MD: Aspen Publishers, Inc.

Ekland, E.S. (1991). Hopelessness. In G. McFarland & M.D. Thomas (Eds.), *Psychiatric mental health nursing* (pp. 278–281). Philadelphia: J.B. Lippincott.

Erickson, H., Tomlin, E., & Swain, M.A. (1983). *Modeling and Role-Modeling—A theory and paradigm for nursing.* Lexington, SC: Pine Press.

Forbes, E.J., & Pekala, R.J. (1993). Psychophysiological effects of several stress management techniques. *Psychological Reports, 72*(1), 19–27.

Holden-Lund, C. (1988). Effects of relaxation with guided imagery on surgical stress and wound healing. *Research in Nursing and Health, 11*(4), 235–244.

Houldin, A.D., McCorkle, R., & Lowery, B.J. (1993). Relaxation training and psychoimmunological status of bereaved spouses. *Cancer Nursing, 16*(1), 47–52.

Hughes, C.P. (1991). Community psychiatric nursing and the depressed elderly. *Journal of Advanced Nursing, 16*(5), 565–572.

Jampolsky G. (1979). *Healing is letting go of fear.* Berkeley: Celestial Books.

Johanson, N. (1991). Effectiveness of a stress management program in reading anxiety and depression in nursing students. *Journal of American College Health, 40*(3), 125–129.

Manson, H., Manderino, M.A., & Johnson, M.T. (1993). Chemotherapy: Thoughts and images of patients with cancer. *Oncology Nurses Forum, 20*(3) 527–531.

North American Nursing Diagnosis Association. (1987). *Taxonomy I with complete diagnoses.* St. Louis: Author.

Petterson, D.R., Questad, K.A., & Boltwood, M.D. (1987). Hypnotherapy as a treatment for pain in patients with burns: Research and clinical observations. *Journal of Burn Care Rehabilitation, 8*(4), 263–268.

Rancour, P. (1991). Guided imagery: Healing when curing is out of the question. *Perspectives in Psychiatric Care, 27*(4), 30–33.

Reeder, D.M. (1991). Cognitive therapy of anger management: Theoretical and practical considerations. *Archives of Psychiatric Nursing, 5*(3), 147–150.

Rees, B.L. (1992). Using relaxation with guided imagery to assist primiparas in achieving maternal role attachment. *Journal of Holistic Nursing, 10*(2), 167–182.

Sims, S.E. (1989). Relaxation training as a technique for helping patients cope with the experience of cancer. *Journal of Advanced Nursing, 12*(5), 583–591.

Spiegel, D., Bloom, J., Kraement, H., & Gottheil, E. (1989). Effect of psychosocial treatment on survival of patients with metastatic breast cancer. *The Lancet, 2*(8668), 888–891.

Stuart, G.W., & Sundeen, S.J. (1991). *Principles and practice of psychiatric nursing* (4th ed.). St. Louis: Mosby Year Book.

Valente, S.M. (1990). Clinical hypnosis with school age children. *Archives of Psychiatric Nursing,* 4(2), 131–136.

Valente, S.M. (1991). Using hypnosis with children for pain management. *Oncology Nurses Forum,* 18(4), 699–704.

Zahourek, R.P. (1982). Hypnosis in nursing practice—emphasis on the "problem patient" who has pain. *Journal of Psychosocial Nursing and Mental Health Services,* 20(3), 13–17.

Zerhusen, J.D., Boyle, K., & Wilson, W. (1991). Out of the darkness: Group cognitive therapy for depressed elderly. *Journal of Psychosocial Nursing and Mental Health Services,* 29(9), 16–21.

4 SPIRITUAL CHALLENGES TO HEALTH AND PEACE

Spirit . . . thought by the Ancients to be a breath or wind, connecting us to the Ultimate, the eternal. Spirit . . . intangible, invisible, yet nonetheless real . . . experienced, especially during moments of spiritual ecstasy and periods of spiritual crisis. Does nursing have a role in promoting, maintaining, or restoring spiritual health? Yes, because spiritual well-being has been noted to be an essential factor in general health (Burkhardt, 1989; Ellison, 1983).

Many nurses have much wisdom and experience in the realm of spiritual care, but avoid or ignore the spiritual dimension, or seek the tangible among the elements composing spirituality. Why this discomfort with the spiritual dimension of care? Perhaps the discomfort lies in the ambiguity, lack of precision, and lack of agreed-on definitions for the concepts underlying spirituality.

THE MEANING OF SPIRITUALITY

Spirituality has been described as "the life principle which pervades and animates a person" (Dombeck & Karl, 1987, p. 184) and "the information nexus which binds things and people and the world together and informs a thing of its nature and context" (Green, 1986, p. 1088). Burkhardt (1991) lists common characteristics of spirituality identified in nursing and other health-related literature:

1. A unifying force within persons
2. A source for discovering and struggling with meaning and purpose in life
3. Relatedness to and connectedness or bonding with all of life, which includes self, others, nature, and frequently God or Higher Power
4. A sense of peace and harmony with the universe
5. Awareness, consciousness, and inner strength. (p. 32)

Major themes identified in this literature suggest that spirituality involves "one's capacity for encountering mystery . . . openness to the transcendent"; "an orientation . . . toward relatedness or connectedness with self, others, nature, and God or Universal Force"; "the deepest core of one's being, the source of inner resources, strength, creativity, and knowledge of oneself" (p. 34).

Furthermore, spirituality is determined to be personal, and yet social and relational (Burkhardt, 1991, p. 34). Stoll (1989) describes spirituality as having both a vertical and a horizontal component, interacting in a continuous interrelationship. The person's inner being interacts in a vertical relationship with the transcendent God or with supreme values that guide the person's life; and in horizontal relationships with self, others, and the environment (pp. 7–8). Factors influencing the individual's relationships with God, self, others, and the environment are grounded in expressions of love, forgiveness, and trust, and the relationships result in meaning and purpose in life (p. 8).

Nurses often experience difficulty differentiating between spirituality, religion, and the psychosocial dimension. It is easier to focus on the more concrete aspects of religious doctrines and rituals rather than on abstract spiritual needs. Additionally, the close association between psychology and nursing has led to difficulty in separating spiritual needs from psychosocial needs.

Spiritual needs have been defined in terms of what is necessary to maintain the vertical and horizontal interrelationships. The essential spiritual need is the need for transcendence. Ellison (1983) defines this need for transcendence to be the need for a sense of well-being experienced when one finds purposes to commit to that involve ultimate meaning for life (p. 330). Both religious and sociopsychological components are involved in spiritual well-being. Associated with the need for transcendence, more specifically described spiritual needs (Highfield & Cason, 1983; Stallwood & Stoll, 1975) include:

1. Forgiveness (from God, self, and others)

2. Unconditional love (given to and received from God, self, and others)

3. Hope and trust

4. Creativity

5. Meaning and purpose in life

Stoll (1989) concludes that the literature describes spirituality to be:

> the vertical dimension of a forgiving, loving, trusting relationship with a God (as defined by that person) and meaningfully lived out in the love, forgiveness, hope, and trust of oneself and others (p. 17).

Figure 4.1 depicts this relationship.

SPIRITUAL WELL-BEING AND HEALTH

Acceptance of a holism paradigm in health care has increased acceptance of the spirit as an essential dimension of health. If there is a body-mind-spirit interaction that cannot be separated into parts, then the spiritual dimension must be interwoven throughout all aspects of life. Unmet spiritual needs can precipitate a physical or emotional illness, and physical or emotional illness can precipitate a spiritual crisis.

EVIDENCE OF SPIRITUAL CRISIS

Distress of the human spirit occurs when spiritual needs are not met. Distress can occur when spiritual needs are unmet in either

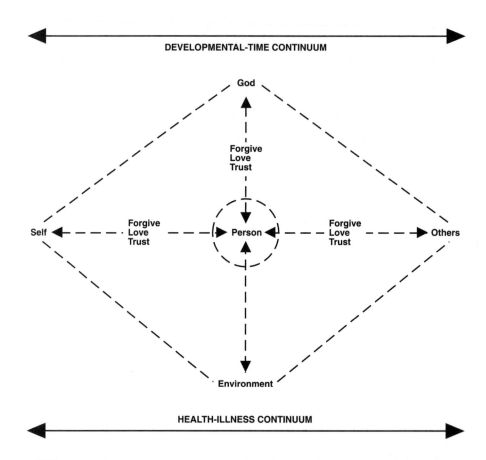

FIGURE 4.1   The person's spiritual interrelatedness. Interrelatedness via forgiveness, love, and trust, resulting in meaning, purpose, and hope in life.
From Stoll, R. (1989). In V.B. Carson, *Spiritual dimensions of nursing practice* (p. 8). Philadelphia: W.B. Saunders. Used with permission.

the religious or existential well-being dimensions, as expressed in the vertical relationship with God or in the horizontal relationships with self and others. Impairment in any of these relationships results in common human responses identified as nursing diagnoses.

The principal nursing diagnosis is spiritual distress (or distress of the human spirit), defined as "a disruption in the life principle that pervades a person's entire being and that integrates and transcends one's biological nature" (NANDA, 1992, p. 46). Persons experiencing spiritual distress may express concerns about meaning or purpose in life, death, and suffering; about conflicts in beliefs and values; and about participation in religious rituals. They may describe hopelessness, describe illness as a punishment, or describe a variety of somatic complaints. They may seek or avoid spiritual assistance. They may exhibit mood and behavioral changes, such as anger, hostility, crying, anxiety, or withdrawal.

Several other NANDA nursing diagnoses are related to spiritual crisis, and others remain to be developed for inclusion in the official list. As can be concluded from the list of spiritual needs, such diagnoses as hopelessness, anxiety/fear, ineffective individual coping, and powerlessness must be considered for clients in spiritual crisis. (See chapter 3 for a discussion of these nursing diagnoses related to mental and emotional crises.) Suggested plans and interventions can be readily adapted for use with clients in spiritual crisis.

Nursing care for spiritual crisis must be based on mutual goal setting with the client. Some nurses find it difficult to avoid proselytizing. The nurse needs to understand the client's world and assist the client to meet personal spiritual goals, support the client's personal beliefs, assist the client to fulfill perceived religious obligations, and promote the client's relationship with a personal deity. The nurse should provide needed spiritual resources that the client cannot obtain without assistance. The nurse should assist the client to find meaning in life and in the current circumstances, to find hope, to increase self-esteem, and to mend disrupted relationships.

By what means can a nurse accomplish such broad and open-ended tasks? The nurse can use active listening and can model the client's world.

PLANNING CARE

The discomfort many caregivers feel when called on to deal with spiritual needs reflects the deeply intimate nature of spirituality. A person's spirituality is so intimately intertwined with a sense of self, a sense of self much broader than what is called self-esteem. Rather, this is the sense of self interrelating with God, others, and all of existence; it is intensely individual, unique.

Because the client is the only one who can experience this intimate sense of her own spirituality, the caregiver must understand the client's model of her spiritual world. The Modeling and Role-Modeling theory is exquisitely suited for providing a framework for spiritual care.

In order to model the client's spiritual world, the nurse must understand that world. Listening and presence, used in their most therapeutic forms, are perhaps the most important nursing tools. Through presence and active listening, a trusting relationship can be established as a basis for exploring the experience of the client's spirituality. Once understood, the client's spiritual world can be modeled by the nurse. This modeling can increase the trust of the relationship so that the client and nurse can work together toward needed interventions.

Spiritual distress can be mild or moderate, more evident of spiritual challenge and an opportunity to grow spiritually. Or, the distress can be so great that the levels of life interruption and intrusion are surpassed, and a sense of encapsulation results. As suggested in the Adaptive Potential Model (see chapter 2), planning for spiritual care depends on assessment of the client's status regarding equilibrium, arousal, or impoverishment. Interventions focus on motivating the client to mobilize available resources, and even in impoverishment, on assisting the client to perceive some level of control.

INTERVENTIONS FOR SPIRITUAL CARE

Nurses are often in the business of solving clients' problems—treating their infection, their cancer; mobilizing their resources to meet physical needs. Spiritual care is not about solving spiritual problems. It is about helping clients to process their feelings, concerns, and thoughts.

Providing spiritual care means being present to the person. Active listening conveys this presence. To minister spiritually to ourselves and to others requires seeing beyond the body, seeing with a deeper vision into the soul of the being that gives that body its life. It is this spirit that longs to be discovered, recognized, and loved in ourselves and in others.

What does it mean to listen? To be listened to? It is to hear the cry of the soul. To hear with trusting love and without judgment. It is through this kind of active listening that nurses can be a channel for expressing God's offer of meaning and purpose, love and relatedness, and forgiveness.

Active listening may involve just listening, touching, or asking questions, exploring feelings behind the content of the words expressed. A simple touch with understanding while listening may begin to establish the trust that is needed for self-revelation. A chaplain once shared that the main tool a minister uses is words. Yet one of his most powerful spiritual experiences occurred when he was asked by a patient to be present with her without using words. In silence and by the holding of hands, the bond of love and relatedness formed through the transcendence of spirit between the minister and the patient. Nurses often do this in their own practice—by smoothing the brow of an anxious client, or holding the hand of someone undergoing a painful or frightening treatment—offering that presence, reassuring the person that he is not alone in his experience. That presence bonds one human being to another.

Unlike ministers, nurses have many tools with which to minister to clients: words of information, pills to ease physical pain, devices and products to ease symptoms of distress. While these tools are valued and needed, the ministering to the inner person through active listening as nurses give shots, pass pills, and address physical wounds may enhance the use of these tools, and at times may decrease the need for them by uncovering the needs that may be the real cause of the symptoms.

Nurses often feel a need to fix what is broken. Instead, we might serve clients better if we simply explored with them their sense of brokenness. From where does it stem? What promotes or diminishes that brokenness? What resources have mended past wounds? Perhaps the greatest ministry is to assist clients to look inside themselves for the answers. For those who believe in Jesus, it may help to remember that He often responded, not by solving problems with answers, but by asking questions or relating parables that the listeners had to work out for themselves.

Questions that are useful in active listening include those that:

1. invite exploration and description (what, how, who, when, where questions):

   "What mood are you feeling today?" rather than "Are you angry?"

   "What are you thinking about at night that keeps you awake?"

   "What is missing or not working in your relationship with God? With your wife?"

   "When did you start feeling that no one loves you?"

   "How have you responded to that feeling?"

2. Ask for sequencing, relating, processing, or reflection:

   "How is your treatment going?" "How do you feel about your treatment?"

   "How have you coped with similar situations in the past?"

   "What were you thinking that triggered the hurt feelings?"

Active listening and presence require commitment, empathy, humility, and an openness to emotional risk, or vulnerability. Spiritual care requires all of these plus an awareness of one's own spirituality. It is not necessary to share a belief system or level of spiritual growth with the client to provide effective spiritual care. But it is essential to have explored one's own spirituality and to recognize one's openness or resistance to varying forms of spiritual expression.

Many clients want to be prayed with or want scripture read to them. Others request participation in religious rituals. The nurse has a responsibility to meet these spiritual needs. If the client's request conflicts with the nurse's values, then the nurse can find others to meet the client's specific needs. In so doing, the nurse must convey acceptance of the client, avoiding the rejection that can so easily be communicated in such circumstances.

CASE STUDY | *Sue*

(This case study is modified from the work of Linda Hunter, MSN, RN, H. Lee Moffit Cancer Center, Tampa, FL. Used with permission.)

Sue, a courageous 32-year-old woman, was diagnosed with advanced sarcoma of the pelvis. She was the wife of a very loving and devoted husband, and the mother of a cherished 6-year-old daughter and 10-year-old son. The aggressiveness of her disease required the surgical removal of the lower half of her body, which included diversion of her bowel and urinary system and removal of her pelvis and legs. At first, most of the nurses caring for Sue could not understand her consent to this extreme, disfiguring, palliative procedure. Yet, her goal was to be rid of the dead part of her body, which was causing so much pain, odor, and immobility, in the hope of increasing the quality of her life for the remainder of her time with her family.

When the nurses met her family and understood the love she had for them, the nurses better understood her desire for the surgery. The surgery was a success in terms of her goal. The time given to her was only six weeks, but in that time Sue found continued meaning and purpose in her life through the love and relatedness she experienced from a husband, children, and nurses who accepted her with two ostomies and half a body. Their acceptance was expressed by their willingness to care for her ostomies . . . lovingly, gently, and expertly, without any outward display of judgment as to her new body image (and Sue looked at each caregiver's face for a reaction to her body!).

Sue found only love and kindness through the nurses' natural ease in relating to her and providing expert care with compassion for her many needs. The nurses initiated a weekly multidisciplinary team conference to present her needs and discuss actions to be taken. Sue participated actively in the decision-making process. She said she felt so much love expressed through the intensive physical and emotional care that she received from the hospital staff. That care consisted of listening and responding to her feelings; seeking help for her and for themselves in understanding and dealing with Sue's feelings and with theirs as well; helping Sue to achieve her goal of pain control; assisting her with life arrangements, and doing it Sue's way to help her maintain a sense of personal control and self-esteem; spending time with Sue sharing laughter, tears, expressions of love; and providing special events, such as "Beauty Parlor Days," promoting her self-esteem by maintaining her femininity with hair shampooing and setting, and nail polishing in her choice of color (usually bright red). Sue's family also expressed feeling loved as the nurses spent many hours with them, allowing time to grieve, to share concerns and their love for Sue.

Each of those whose lives she touched in turn received from her added meaning and purpose in their own lives. A nurse told of a change in priorities within her own family life. An ostomy volunteer, who gave encouragement and acceptance to Sue through the sharing of their mutual experiences of ostomies and cancer's life threat, told of the impact of Sue's courageous friendship.

The ostomy visitor was the channel through which Sue developed a deep spiritual communion with the hospital chaplain. Not knowing that Sue had refused to see a chaplain because of some past negative experience with a minister, the ostomy volunteer asked her minister to visit Sue. When she shared this with the nurse, the nurse asked Sue if she wanted her to tell him not to come. Because of her trust in her friendship with the ostomy visitor, Sue allowed the minister to visit. That visit paved the way for the hospital chaplain to begin to minister to Sue—a ministry that bonded her relationship with God and which she described to be a source of great peace for her.

Once Sue thanked a nurse for her spiritual care. When asked how Sue thought the nurse had given her spiritual care, Sue said that the nurse had heard her, had understood what she meant when she talked, had asked questions to clarify so that the nurse really understood her needs. She said that so many people listen but don't really hear. She added that the nurse had given her skillful, competent care, delivered with compassion for her total well-being. Sue noted the extra time that nurse would take unblocking her colostomy or staying beyond her shift to be with Sue's family during an emergency surgery.

When Sue's body finally died, the loving, humorous, kind spirit lived on. It is that spirit that lives on in eternity and through the lives of the people who were privileged to care for her and be cared about by her. We told many of the staff that she found meaning in her suffering through all the loving relationships she had formed while in their care. The day Sue died, she asked her hospice nurse if today was the day. The nurse asked what she meant. Sue said, "Is this the day I'm going to die?" The nurse said she didn't know, but that it might be the day. Sue spent the remainder of her conscious hours completing her unfinished business—writing a letter to her children and husband, sharing with them once again her love for them, instructing the funeral home director about last thoughts on her funeral.

The week after the funeral, the staff had a memorial service at the hospital. Her family and all who cared for her were present. At the service, each person had an opportunity to share with Sue's family and each other the meaning, purpose, and love that each had gained from having cared for Sue. They were able to express to each other the bonds that were formed among all of them because of the opportunity her care provided for sharing the gifts each gave to and received from her and from each other.

Purpose is a precious blueprint which, when well defined, gives life direction and meaning. It synergies all life activities. Sue found purpose in her life until the moment of her death.

Discussion

The essential component of spiritual care is seeing and experiencing the client's world. Sue required so much physical care that it would have been easy to lose any sense of the person behind the care needs. Her disfigurement could easily have produced revulsion in caregivers, and the revulsion could have resulted in avoidance. Nurses who do not analyze their own feelings or who do not see the client holistically tend to construct a care plan full of physically related nursing diagnoses and collaborative problems, possibly missing the nursing diagnoses most essential to Sue's well-being.

Holistic nurses caring for Sue were able to see the person behind the cancer, the disfigurement. They were

Nursing Diagnosis	Goal	Intervention
High risk for spiritual distress r/t major body disfigurement, increasing pain, past negative experience with a minister, refusal to see chaplain, and impending death	Client will verbalize continued sense of meaning and purpose in life; meaningful relationships with significant others and with God (as defined by pt); and hope.	1. Use active listening to encourage client to express feelings about meaning and purpose, relationships, and religious ritual needs. 2. Attempt to understand the client's view of spirituality and religion. 3. Support client's sense of spirituality. Avoid proselytizing. 4. Offer prayer, read scripture, and other religious measures as appropriate. 5. Provide expert physical care, communicating that client is a valuable individual.
High risk for powerlessness r/t major surgical trauma and body disfigurement, increasing pain, and impending death	Client will verbalize a sense of control.	1. Allow and encourage client to make decisions regarding care: i.e., acceptance or rejection of interventions; timing of care. 2. Teach client details of pain management protocol and work with client to determine pain relief intervention and medication dosage. 3. Validate expression of feelings by encouraging client to talk and using active listening.
High risk for social isolation	Client will describe a sense of being cared for by family and staff.	1. Promote social interactions with family, visitors, and staff. 2. Assist client to dress in clean, becoming clothes or gown, with makeup, hair combed each day to the level allowed by her energy reserves. 3. Maintain clean, neat, attractive environment. 4. Provide adequate pain control. 5. Space social interactions according to energy levels and client's comfort.
Body image disturbance r/t major body disfigurement	Client will describe herself as a whole person even with much of body removed. Client will verbalize and demonstrate acceptance of appearance. Client will participate in self-care of stomas. Client will maintain social contact with others.	1. Avoid any evidence of revulsion when providing care. 2. Encourage client to express feelings about body changes and effect on self-esteem. 3. Promote social interactions. 4. Promote sense of individuality and femininity through continued attention to personal care and beauty measures.
Chronic pain r/t tissue destruction secondary to metastatic cancer	Client's pain will be controlled with few signs of impaired cognition.	1. Monitor pain level, respirations, and cognition. 2. Adjust pain medication to control pain. 3. Administer Therapeutic Touch.
Opportunity to enhance effective grieving RT loss of body parts	See chapter 6.	
Opportunity to enhance anticipatory grieving RT impending death	See chapter 6.	

TABLE 4.1 Nursing Care Plan: Sue

able to see the spirit, the indomitable spirit, and support and encourage Sue's spiritual well-being. Physical care was not neglected, but carried out in a very professional, competent manner, thereby enhancing Sue's sense of value. In addition, the nurses were present and through active listening assisted Sue to a level of transcendence to spiritually surmount the circumstances, to enhance her perception of meaning and purpose, and to deepen her relationships with self, family, and God.

SUMMARY

When nurses understand what is required of them to give effective, competent spiritual care, the reluctance to address the spiritual dimension is overcome. This chapter clarifies both the meaning of spirituality and the nurse's role in spiritual care. By viewing spirituality from a broader perspective than religious practice, the nurse can recognize the many interacting facets that compose spirituality, such as unifying force, meaning and purpose, relatedness and connectedness, and vertical and horizontal relationships.

Assessing and understanding the client's experience of these many facets of spirituality help the nurse determine where care is needed and what care is needed. In spiritual care more than in any other care, the nurse must understand and model the client's world. Active listening, hearing with trusting love and without judgment, is the most essential care component. Another essential component is awareness of one's own spirituality, recognizing openness or resistance to various forms of spiritual expression. Through skillful use of self or, more precisely, use of presence, active listening, and response to specific needs, the nurse can support the client's movement toward transcendence, enhanced perception of meaning and purpose, deepened relationships, and general spiritual well-being.

References

Burkhardt, M. (1991). Spirituality and children: Nursing considerations. *Journal of Holistic Nursing, 9*(2), 31–40.

Burkhardt, M. (1989). Spirituality: An analysis of the concept. *Holistic Nursing Practice, 3*(3), 69–77.

Dombeck, M., & Karl, J. (1987). Spiritual issues in mental health. *Journal of Religion and Health, 26*(3), 183–197.

Ellison, C. (1983). Spiritual well-being: Conceptualization and measurement. *Journal of Psychology and Theology, 11*(4), 330–340.

Green, R. (1986). Healing and spirituality. *The Practitioner, 1422*(230), 1087–1093.

Highfield, M., & Cason, C. (1983). Spiritual needs of patients: Are they recognized? *Cancer Nursing, 6*(3), 187–192.

North American Nursing Diagnosis Association (NANDA). (1992). *Nursing diagnosis: Definitions and classification.* Philadelphia: Author.

Stallwood, J., & Stoll, R. (1975). Spiritual dimension of nursing practice. In I. Beland & J. Passos (Eds.), *Clinical nursing* (3rd ed.) (pp. 1086–1098). New York: Macmillan.

Stoll, R.I. (1989). The essence of spirituality. In V. B. Carson, *Spiritual dimensions of nursing practice* (pp. 4–23). Philadelphia: W. B. Saunders.

Suggested Reading

Charnes, L. S., & Moore, P. S. (1992). Meeting patients' spiritual needs. The Jewish perspective. *Holistic Nursing Practice, 6*(3), 64–72.

Fish, S., & Shelley, J. (1978). *Spiritual care: The nurse's role.* Downers Grove, IL: Intervarsity Press.

Hill, L., & Smith, N. (1985). *Self-care nursing: Promotion of health.* Englewood Cliffs, NJ: Prentice-Hall, Inc.

Mansen, T. (1993). The spiritual dimension of individuals: Conceptual development. *Nursing Diagnosis, 4*(4), 140–147.

Reed, P. (1991). Spirituality and mental health in older adults: Extant knowledge for nursing. *Family and Community Health, 14*(2), 14–25.

Taylor, P., & Ferszt, G. (1990). Spiritual healing. *Holistic Nursing Practice, 4*(4), 32–38.

SPECIAL
CLIENT
SITUATIONS

5 | THE DYING CLIENT

Health care providers are often called upon to provide care to dying clients. But the words *health care* imply healing. Is it reasonable to expect that healing can occur in individuals who are dying? The authors contend that it is. The process of dying can produce great opportunities for personal growth, resulting in a sense of wholeness, of spiritual and emotional well-being. Nurses can have an essential role in bringing about the necessary healing for the dying person to achieve this integrated wholeness.

FACING DEATH AS ONE OF LIFE'S CRISES

Unless death is sudden, the process of dying occurs in stages, and each stage presents opportunities for experiencing crisis. Each crisis of dying can be viewed as a "turning point" (*Webster's*, 1982), when one is "confronted with an unfamiliar obstacle in life's path" (Cunningham, 1991). When "coping responses to stress fail, the event is experienced as overwhelming" (Berger & Williams, 1992). This sense of being overwhelmed can occur at the diagnosis of a disease perceived to be life-threatening, during the course of the illness as physical challenges are confronted, and during the terminal stage when death is near.

Dying is a natural occurrence as one moves through life, and thus it is a maturational crisis. But dying also poses a threat to the individual's steady state, and thereby creates situational crises (see chapter 1). The uniqueness of each person—his history of physical, emotional, and spiritual experiences—makes each individual's response to crises quite personal. It has been suggested that most people handle dying in the same manner in which they usually handle other crises (Callanan & Kelley, 1992, p. 58).

In some respects, death is the ultimate loss—loss of self, and loss of all relationships with other humans and with existence as we know it. But can the losses and crises posed by dying produce anything positive? "Yes!" assert many nurses working with dying patients and their families.

Dying is a time of healing without curing, of healing the soul or inner life and not the body; a time to participate in the conscious process of leave-taking (Schroeder-Sheker, 1993); a time when great personal growth can take place; a parallel to birthing as one makes the transition through death to what lies beyond (Callanan & Kelley, 1992). It can be seen, then, that the dying process can be approached as a series of challenges, requiring special effort and dedication to live life until one dies, and to arrive at death an integrated, whole being.

PHYSICAL CHALLENGES OF DYING

The holistic model presented in chapter 1 emphasizes the interconnectedness of body, mind, and spirit. This interconnection is probably never more evident than during the process of dying. However, the physical challenges associated with dying are unique and will be addressed as separate from other considerations of caring for the dying client.

Terminal illnesses and associated medical treatments are often accompanied by debilitating and extremely distressing symptoms. Physical pain can be excruciating, and its amelioration is a major focus of palliative care. However, it is not unusual for pain to be absent. Nausea, severe constipation or diarrhea, marked debilitation, and fatigue are among the symptoms most likely to provoke crisis responses in dying patients. Taste changes, mucous membrane dryness and lesions, and a decreased interest in food result in weight loss and general debilitation. However, the health and age of the person, the progression of the terminal disease, side effects of related medical treatments, and which organs are involved affect the physical symptoms experienced. Onset of distressing symptoms may be early in the disease process or delayed until nearing death. Death itself may occur while the individual is still alert and aware, or while the person is asleep or in a coma.

Specific physical changes tend to be present when death is near. Callanan and Kelley (1992, pp. 36–39) describe these physical signs. There is difficulty swallowing. Decreased desire for food and fluids may be reinforced by this swallowing difficulty. Mucus may gather in the throat, producing a rattling sound that may or may not be accompanied by difficulty breathing. Breathing may become irregular and periods of apnea or Cheyne-Stokes respirations may occur. Body temperature may rise while hands and feet cool, become mottled or cyanotic. Profuse sweating may occur. Bowel and bladder function decrease and urine becomes darker. As weakness progresses, incontinence may occur, verbal communication becomes minimal and more subtle, and the person may appear to be in a state between sleep and waking, with glazed eyes that remain half open. Hearing remains intact as the last sense to fade. The cessation of breathing is the most obvious sign that death has occurred. The final breaths may be sighs, or a pattern change with longer periods of apnea, or just a gentle slowing to periodic shallow breaths.

All of the concepts presented in chapter 2 concerning the challenges presented by physical illness are relevant to coping with the distressing symptoms of terminal illness. Life patterns are interrupted and change is demanded. With terminal illness, there is the added dimension of ultimate loss. As with other physical illness, terminal illness often is seen as a time for reflection and change. For nurses to support their dying clients, it is important to understand the client's perspective as each stage of the dying process is experienced. Because of the broad-based effect of terminal illness on the surrounding community of family, friends, and others close to the dying person, the nurse using the Modeling and Role-Modeling theory must assist those involved to understand the client's perspective.

THE EXPERIENCE OF DYING

The experience of dying has been examined from many perspectives. Three of these perspectives that are relevant to nurses
planning care for dying clients are stages of the dying process,
the role of hope in reaching a final sense of acceptance and
peace, and the newly described finding of what has been called
"nearing death awareness" (Callanan & Kelley, 1992).

Stages of Dying

Early studies of patients' experiences of dying, such as those of Dr.
Kubler-Ross (1969), described the reactions to dying as occurring
in five stages: denial, anger, bargaining, depression, and acceptance. Ongoing study of the dying experience has revealed that
these reactions do not occur in a specific order, rather they occur
in a shifting, overlapping manner with fluctuation. The reactions
are prompted by the tasks associated with dying. These tasks
include accepting the reality of the diagnosis, adjusting to life with
illness, and preparing for approaching death. Each of these tasks
can and often does produce a crisis for the individual.

Denial serves to protect one from overwhelming pain, and
as a coping strategy it can be beneficial. Fear, helplessness, and
resentment are usual sources of anger, which may be directed at
family and friends closest to the person, at caregivers, organizations, or God. Bargaining serves to provide some hope by post-
poning the inevitable. Depression is a usual reaction associated
with grieving. The losses accompanying dying are many. There
are the losses caused by the illness, and then the losses caused
by death itself, including relationships and the entire future. The
depression provoked by such losses is a natural part of the grieving process. Acceptance may or may not occur, but if so, it usually occurs very near death. Acceptance is reflected in peaceful
resignation and detaching from persons and events of this world.

The Role of Hope: Meeting the Challenge

Two recent studies have examined the experience of hope and
of health in the terminally ill. Hall (1990) noted that hope in the

presence of terminal illness has been viewed by some to be unrealistic and evidence of denial, and by others as essential to maintaining emotional well-being in any circumstances. Exploring the concept of hope as it is lived by persons with terminal illness, Hall found hope to mean:

1. having a future life in spite of the diagnosis,

2. having a renewed zest for life,

3. finding reason for living, usually one not evident before, and

4. finding a treatment believed to contribute to survival. (p. 183)

Fryback (1993) studied how health was described by persons diagnosed with potentially terminal diseases, and how these persons applied the concept of health to themselves. Three domains of health emerged from the data: mental/emotional, spiritual, and physical. Key concepts within the mental/emotional domain included hope, love, and control. The spiritual domain included belief in a higher power, recognition of mortality, and self-actualization. Health in the physical domain included health promotion activities, feeling good, and a relationship with the physician.

Informants in this study also identified hope as an essential component of health. What informants perceived to be unhealthy was not having a diagnosed disease, but being unable to live life fully or to do desired things. Many informants had made changes in their lives that produced a sense of greater peace and happiness, and, thereby, a healthier state even in the presence of the diagnosed disease.

These studies suggest that the crises experienced in dying can be reframed as challenges. The challenges can be met through means that inspire hope and a sense of health even in the presence of terminal illness.

Nearing Death

Recent studies have begun to examine the experiences of persons nearing death, their attempts to describe and communicate these experiences, and to determine what is needed to make their death a peaceful one. Schroeder-Sheker (1993) describes the process of dying in terms of *rite of passage*. Callanan and Kelley (1992) present a description of Nearing Death Awareness, a theory relating to the experiences of persons dying slowly, as opposed to those near-death experiences reported by persons who are resuscitated after clinical death.

The anthropological term *rite of passage* conveys a meaning of transformation, of transition from one culturally based life state/role to another. Applied to the dying process (Turner, 1975; Van Gennep, 1961), three stages are identified: the rites of separation, the rites of liminality, and the rites of reincorporation. During the liminal (or threshold) period, bonds loosen and structural relationships and classifications become obscure, and the person is in a state unlike either the known of earthly existence or the coming state of death. It is during this liminal state that specific types of music can "help the body and soul unbind (not destroy) the threads that sustain life processes by freeing patients from time" (Schroeder-Sheker, 1993, p. 44). Studies of patient responses to such music have shown that some patients drift into deep sleep and find a level of relief from suffering not achieved by morphine (p. 44).

Callanan and Kelley (1992) define Nearing Death Awareness as "a special knowledge about—and sometimes a control over—the process of dying" (p. 13). Dying persons communicate, often with symbolic language and potent metaphors, descriptions of what dying is like and what they need to die peacefully. Because the experiences described often contain glimpses of another world and visions of loved ones or spiritual beings who are waiting in that world, family members and caregivers mistake the descriptions for confusion, dementia, or delirium. When asked to describe what they are seeing, the dying frequently say that there are no words to describe the beauty and intensity. Commonly described feelings include warmth, peace, and feeling loved; an absence of fear, but a concern for loved ones being left behind (p. 16). The dying often know that they are dying whether or not they have been told, and often communicate in advance the time when they will die (p. 15).

Requests regarding needs to make a death peaceful are often expressed in symbolic language and may be difficult to decipher (Callanan & Kelley, 1992, p. 15). Such requests usually involve others, such as requests for assistance with healing relationships, meeting with someone, or remaining alive for a meaningful event. The dying seem to be able to control the time and circumstances of their death in order for these needs to be met.

PLANNING CARE

The Modeling and Role-Modeling theory (Erickson, Tomlin, & Swain, 1983) is exquisitely suited to care of the dying (see chapter 1). The basis for this theory is understanding the client's model of his world, communicating this to the client, and mutually setting goals for care. Because each individual is unique, each has a unique model of the world, and of dying. As noted by Callanan and Kelley (1992), most caregivers are not yet aware of what dying persons are trying to communicate about their nearing death experiences. Furthermore, the dying have a need for caregivers to foster hope and a sense of health even during the dying process. In order to meet these varied needs, nurses must learn to model the client's world.

Nursing interventions may be needed at various stages of the dying process; during the initial period of diagnosis of terminal illness, during the progression of the illness, or during the nearing death period. Individualized interventions based on the client's model of the world at any given stage are guided by the five aims of intervention (see chapter 1). Efforts to model the client's world help to build trust and to establish a positive nurse-client relationship. The nurse must attend to physical as well as psychosocial needs associated with dying, determining interventions based on the client's priorities.

The level of interruption, intrusion, or sense of encapsulation felt by the client during the stages of dying varies with the stage and with the individual. Use of Bowman's (1992) guide to the Adaptive Potential Model (see chapter 2) can help to base interventions on the client's state of equilibrium, arousal, or impoverishment. When the client is in adaptive equilibrium, the nurse can support client efforts and coping strategies. When maladaptive equilibrium is assessed, the nurse can motivate change by helping the client to identify and mobilize coping resources or by providing direct care if the client is in impoverishment. Assisting the client to perceive control over as much of life and life processes as possible is an essential component of care for the dying.

Nursing Interventions

Nursing interventions for the client in the various stages of dying should be based on the combined understanding of the client's model of her world and the utility of the reactions as coping mechanisms. Callanan and Kelley (1992) speak to the most effective approaches. Denial should not be challenged. The nurse should neither reinforce nor encourage denial, nor use false cheer to overcome it. It is not the nurse's role to make the client accept reality. The nurse should use responses that acknowledge hopes and wishes but do not reinforce the denial being communicated. When anger is expressed, look for the cause, and try to avoid feeling personally attacked. Avoid trying to talk the person out of anger. This may only intensify the anger. If the helplessness or fear underlying the anger can be addressed, the anger may abate. If bargaining is described, treat it as suggested for denial. Make comments that acknowledge the desire for what is being bargained for. Avoid lecturing the client on the improbability of the bargaining working. It seems that some dynamic in bargaining often does work, such as living until a particular event occurs. Feelings of depression should be honored rather than dismissed or downplayed. Listening is the primary skill needed, along with an attempt to understand the feelings. When a client reaches a stage of acceptance, there is a drawing away from others. Encourage the presence of one or two significant people, and help them to understand that the drawing away process is a natural part of dying and not a rejection of them.

The greatest skills needed to support a client in the various stages of dying are attentive listening and accepting the client at the particular point in the process. Another aspect of care is the ability to accept the expression of pain, and to accept the pain that the nurse will feel, without trying to say or do something to avoid the pain and sadness.

Care for Those Nearing Death

Beyond immediate physical care and pain control, the nurse has a major role in caring for clients nearing death. The focus of this care is facilitating communication between the client and significant others. A major focus of this role is teaching friends and family how to listen, understand, and respond appropriately to the symbolic or cryptic messages of the dying loved one (Callanan & Kelley, 1992, pp. 241–246). The following suggestions, which are presented for the caregivers, especially family or friends, are equally useful for nurses caring for dying clients.

1. Pay attention to *everything* the dying person says, and write notes on gestures, conversations, and out-of-the-ordinary communications. Discuss the notes with others to help to identify clues of meaning.
2. Be alert for important messages in *any* communication, even if vague or garbled.
3. Watch for signs that the person is experiencing something not of this world: glassy-eyed look; staring through you; distractedness or secretiveness; inappropriate smiles or gestures, such as pointing, reaching toward something visible only to the dying person, waving; picking at the covers; attempts to get out of bed for no apparent reason; agitation or distress at others' inability to comprehend something the dying person is trying to say.
4. Use gentle inquiries to clarify what you don't understand: "Can you tell me what is happening?"
5. Use open-ended, encouraging questions to clarify what the dying person is trying to communicate about what is being experienced. If the person is describing seeing someone long dead, confirm the comfort that the experience must provide, and ask, "Can you tell me more?"
6. Accept and validate what the dying person tells you.
7. Don't argue or challenge.
8. Be alert to the use of images from life experiences like work or hobbies.
9. Be honest about having trouble understanding.
10. Don't push. Let the dying control the breadth and depth of the conversation.
11. Avoid instilling a sense of failure in the dying person. Appreciate the effort made to communicate even if the message is garbled or vague.

12. If you don't know what to say, don't say anything.

13. Be alert to the fact that the dying often try to communicate important information to someone who makes them feel safe, who may be an outsider. This person must share the information with those most likely to note the innuendos in a message. (pp. 241–243)

In all of the communications by the dying person, all caregivers and significant people should be aware that the content of the messages may fall into categories of what is being experienced, what is needed to die peacefully, and the timing of death. A further pattern of communication related to dying peacefully and timing of death is a communication about something holding the person back (p. 244). Once the meaning of the communication is clear, communicate this understanding to the dying person, and let the person know that you are working on the issue at hand.

MUSIC THANATOLOGY

A creative use of music as therapy is emerging for assisting the dying with the transition from life to death. This use of music is called *music thanatology* (Schroeder-Sheker, 1993). Based on the use of music and the concepts of spirituality, sacredness, and beauty developed by the Cluny monks of the tenth century, music thanatology uses "sound anointings" (p. 42) to "*unbind* or *loosen* a patient from what it is that binds one so deeply to the physical body" (p. 44). The primary goals of this use of music as a deathbed vigil are comfort and a peaceful and conscious death. Anecdotal evidence and beginning research findings support a remarkable effect on pain relief and agitation. The pain relief reported is greater than that achieved by narcotic analgesics. Thus, music thanatology promotes peacefulness at the time of death.

NURSING DIAGNOSIS

Nurses providing care to dying clients express nursing concerns in the diagnostic language of nursing diagnosis. As with physical illness, physiologically based nursing diagnoses are readily established. Those diagnoses associated with the emotional responses to the dying process require more refined and sensitive critical thought. During the stage of terminal illness diagnosis and early disease process, assessment focuses on the client's adaptive equilibrium. Identified maladaptive equilibrium may generate such nursing diagnoses as anxiety, fear, social isolation, and ineffective individual coping. Later in the process, many nursing diagnoses, such as spiritual distress, spiritual well-being, powerlessness, or hopelessness, may be identified; they may also involve caregivers, caregiver role strain, and compromised family coping. Identifying and intervening for nursing diagnoses in the mental/emotional/spiritual domain in a manner that enhances the person's sense of hope, love, and control can result in a dying client's perceiving a state of health, even as the dying process progresses to death (Fryback, 1993).

CASE STUDY | *Mr. Lin*

(Adapted from the work of Lola Lehman, 1993. Used with permission.)

Mr. Lin was a 60-year-old man who was married and had three daughters living in the same community. He was retired from a local printing agency where he had established a reputation for his conscientious and meticulous creations.

Several years of illness had forced Mr. Lin to retire early, and soon after retirement he was diagnosed with lung cancer. His symptoms had been treated for several years. He was experiencing progressively more pain, requiring more and more aggressive treatment with medications. Mr. Lin was referred to a hospice agency when the illness became advanced, with a life expectancy of approximately six months.

The client and family were very receptive to the hospice nurse, David. During the first visit, Mr. Lin's wife and daughters were present. They had all accepted, at varying levels, that they were dealing with a terminal illness. It was evident that this crisis was a family affair. They all wanted to be involved and wanted information about how to best help the client.

David spent time orienting the client and family to the hospice services, allowed them to vent their concerns and feelings, and encouraged them to identify their needs. Some of the family's questions were asked outside the range of the client's hearing. The family was in a state of arousal and needed help mobilizing their resources. David planned to provide support for them so that they could continue their supportive care of the client. Rapport and trust were easily established with this family.

To establish trust with the client, David encouraged him to talk about his illness. Mr. Lin was very articulate about the effect of the illness. He described the interruption in his retirement plans to pursue his musical interests. He had purchased a piano. He was very angry about the failure of the medical profession to diagnose his condition earlier. Pain and fatigue were intruding on his activities, and he was confining himself to the house, mostly watching TV and reading. His wife had been taking him for rides, but frightening episodes of shortness of breath on exertion made him confine himself to the house. He acknowledged that he had difficulty letting others, including his wife, help him, preferring to do things by himself even when this caused increased exertion.

Mr. Lin perceived his illness to be encapsulating. His main focus was on his pain, his fatigue, and fear about his spiritual life. Concerns that he expressed included: "having pain and feeling so tired that I don't enjoy doing the things I used to do or had planned to do"; "making me feel less like a man"; "not able to care for my family"; "worrying that I have waited too late to make my peace with God."

To focus holistically on this client, the nurse considered the mind, body, and spirit. Nursing care of the body focused on controlling the pain; nursing care of the mind focused on assisting Mr. Lin and his family to move toward acceptance of death; and nursing care of the spirit focused on dealing with his spiritual concerns. Meeting these needs would enhance the probability of his attaining a peaceful death. The plan was designed to maintain a balance between the three areas of body, mind, and spirit because a dysfunction in one area directly affects the other areas.

The five principles of intervention were incorporated into the plan. Trust was established by being open and receptive to Mr. Lin, allowing him to express his feelings without interruption. Open-ended questions were used to further encourage him to express his thoughts and feelings. David communicated acceptance of Mr. Lin's feelings throughout the relationship.

As Mr. Lin moved toward death, David sought to help him identify areas of strength and maintain a sense of control. Interventions focused on three areas identified to be of major concern to the client: his pain, his spiritual distress, and his changing relationship with his wife.

As the pain increased, the medication had to be regulated continually. The medication was regulated to provide comfort at a level that prevented severe cognitive change. The pain control improved Mr. Lin's quality of life, allowing him to continue to interact with his loved ones.

Initially, Mr. Lin expressed greatest concern about his relationship with his God. He had no denominational affiliation, but he was a Christian. David was comfortable in the role of spiritual counselor, but Mr. Lin viewed David as a nurse and had difficulty accepting his nurse in both roles. The hospice agency provided a ministerial counselor who provided great support for Mr. Lin. Mr. Lin identified that prayer was helpful to him, and David began to pray with him each visit just before leaving. David used short, three- or four-sentence prayers focused on the client's problems. One response was, "That's just what I need. Thanks for not including all the world problems." The content of the prayers changed as Mr. Lin's condition changed, initially focusing on strength, then control of pain, and then acceptance of death— "as he walks through the valley of the shadow of death continue to comfort him so he has no need to fear." Gradually the client was able to resolve his spiritual concerns and began to talk more openly about death and a sense of preparation.

Mr. Lin gradually became less interested in socialization. He perceived his wife to be angry because he was interfering with her social activities. She was a very social individual and was involved in numerous activities, many of which she had to give up in order to care for him. He felt that his wife was moving away from him, not loving him as she had. He was missing their intimacy. David encouraged him to talk to his wife about his feelings. The nurse discussed with the client the behavior of terminally ill clients and their loved ones, especially the pattern of withdrawing from each other as a means of self-preservation. The suggestion was made that perhaps Mr. Lin was also withdrawing from his wife. Mr. Lin reported that he talked with his wife and stated, "There is not enough loving going on here and it has to stop." His wife understood his feelings and regained her affectionate manner. This helped Mr. Lin to regain some sense of control and enhanced his self-esteem. David suggested that Mrs. Lin use respite care so that she could continue some of her social activities while assuring that her husband was being provided skillful care.

When Mr. Lin became very weak and began falling, David talked with Mrs. Lin about a hospital bed. Mr. Lin was very depressed on the next visit. He stated that he was not prepared for the bed. It presented reality. He had begun to accept his death intellectually; however, he had not begun to accept it emotionally. The bed had forced him to sense the finality of his situation. David should have prepared him for the change and involved him in the decision to help him maintain a sense of control. In this instance, David had failed to model the client's world.

Mr. Lin had a wonderful sense of humor which he maintained throughout the illness. It was not a cover-up. It was a means for him to take a minirest from his serious business of dying. It was his affirmation of life at a time when he perceived others to be treating him as already dead. That sense of humor was a source of comfort for the family. It allowed them a release of tension.

David helped Mr. Lin maintain hope throughout the experience. He was not denied the opportunity to dream. At first his dreams were extravagant, such as writing a book. As his disease progressed and his strength decreased, his dreams became smaller. With unrealistic dreams, David would comment, "I don't know if you will be able to do that or not, but I sure hope that you can."

On David's second-to-last visit, Mr. Lin summarized the relationship. When David left, he felt as if it were Mr. Lin's way of saying goodbye—a nearing death awareness. David did not expect to see him the next week. He talked with the family about letting go, of giving Mr. Lin permission to die. The family continued to reassure Mr. Lin of their love and of the fact that they would manage and would take care of each other.

By the next week, the client's lungs were filling with fluid. The oldest daughter had learned to use a suction machine. Mr. Lin drifted in and out of consciousness. During more lucid periods, David talked to him about all the artistic designs the client had made in his lifetime and how they could be found throughout the country. David acknowledged the time and energy that Mr. Lin had devoted to each design. Mr. Lin's breathing was shallow. The family called David aside and asked what they could expect, how would they know when death had occurred. David explained about Cheyne-Stokes respirations and other physical symptoms. Before leaving, David noticed that Mr. Lin's respirations were slowing. He leaned over and said, "Goodbye." Mr. Lin responded, "Goodbye," and in less than ten minutes he died. Mr. Lin's death was truly peaceful. He died with dignity.

David had left the house minutes before Mr. Lin died. As soon as David was notified, he returned to the home. The daughter shared her appreciation for the information about what to expect. The daughter stated that the death had occurred just as David had told them it would. David complimented Mrs. Lin and the daughters on their care. They were comforted by knowing that they had done all they could.

Nursing Diagnosis	Goal	Intervention
Activity intolerance r/t pain and weakness/fatigue	Client will be able to participate in one planned activity per day.	1. Assess level of weakness regularly. 2. Encourage balance of rest and activity. 3. Identify times of greatest strength and encourage activities at those times.
Caregiver role strain r/t uncertainty about duration and extent of caregiving required	Caregiver will exhibit few signs of stress such as irritability towards patient or care he requires.	1. Encourage expression of feelings. 2. Provide knowledge. 3. Provide and encourage use of hospice volunteer and respite worker.
Grieving r/t impending death	Client will verbalize acceptance of death.	1. Assess stage. 2. Support at that stage. 3. Encourage verbalization of feelings.
Powerlessness r/t decreasing ability as death approaches	Client will verbalize that he feels a sense of some control.	1. Include in decision making. 2. Maintain hope. 3. Raise self-esteem. 4. Maintain humor.
Spiritual distress r/t uncertainty about relationship with God	Client will verbalize his fear about dying.	1. Encourage to discuss feelings, identify religious orientation. 2. Refer for religious counseling. 3. Identify helpful measures. 4. Offer prayer or other appropriate measures.
Pain, chronic r/t physiology of illness	Client's pain will be controlled with few signs of impaired cognition.	1. Assess pain level. 2. Regulate medication to control. 3. Administer Therapeutic Touch.
Social isolation r/t caregivers not understanding meanings of nearing death communication pattern	Caregivers will encourage and communicate acceptance of client's description of the dying experience, including conversations with deceased persons, out-of-body experiences, and statements regarding probable time of death.	1. Communicate acceptance of client's descriptions of nearing death experiences. 2. Assist family to understand nearing death communication patterns, including mutual withdrawal, client's decreasing verbal communication, cryptic messages about experiences of dying, meaning of perceived encounters with deceased or spiritual beings.

TABLE 5.1   *Nursing Care Plan: Mr. Lin*

Discussion

Accepting the client's view of his world is an essential part of Modeling and Role-Modeling theory. It is this acceptance and validation of the client's experiences that keep open the communication with caregivers, especially with dying clients whose experiences may not be readily understood by those who are not dying. Caregivers who maintain open communication and model the client's world help the client maintain a sense of control. The one breach of this modeling, when the nurse sought to meet the wife's need for a hospital bed to assist with her caregiving, pushed the client into a crisis state. Acceptance of Mr. Lin's open communication of this crisis state helped the wife and the nurse to again model the client's world and return to a far more therapeutic pattern of interaction with him, resulting in his peaceful death.

SUMMARY

Nurses do, indeed, have a role of healing in caring for dying clients. By understanding the client's world, the nurse can recognize what events or circumstances are experienced as crises and can help the dying person mobilize resources to meet the challenges, be they physical, emotional, or spiritual. The nurse's holistic care of the client's mind, body, and spirit becomes clearly focused when the nurse first seeks to understand the client's world; assesses the level of intrusion or encapsulation, and the client's state of equilibrium, arousal, or impoverishment; and formulates relevant nursing diagnoses as a basis for care.

In addition to providing skillful care for the physical needs of dying, the nurse can support the client's and family's needs for a sense of control and self-esteem. Providing accurate information about elements of the dying process and clarifying communications can help to maintain that sense of control and to reinforce a sense of hope. Knowledge of nearing death communication patterns and such innovative therapies as music thanatology can help the client arrive at death an integrated, whole being.

References

Berger, K.J., & Williams, M.B. (1992). *Fundamentals of nursing.* Norwalk, CT: Appleton & Lange.

Bowman, S. (1992, October). *Adaptive potential as a guide to planning nursing interventions.* Presented at the Fourth National Modeling and Role-Modeling Conference, Boston, MA.

Callanan, M., & Kelley, P. (1992). *Final gifts.* New York: Bantam Books.

Cunningham, J.M. (1991). Crisis intervention. In G. McFarland & M.D. Thomas (Eds.), *Psychiatric mental health nursing* (pp. 759–765). Philadelphia: J.B. Lippincott.

Erickson, H., Tomlin, E., & Swain, M.A. (1983). *Modeling and Role-Modeling: A theory and paradigm for nursing.* Lexington, SC: Pine Press.

Fryback, P.B. (1993). Health for people with a terminal diagnosis. *Nursing Science Quarterly, 6*(3), 147–159.

Hall, B.A. (1990). The struggle of the diagnosed terminally ill person to maintain hope. *Nursing Science Quarterly, 3,* 177–184.

Kubler-Ross, E. (1969). *On death and dying.* New York: Macmillan.

Schroeder-Sheker, T. (1993). Music for the dying: A personal account of the new field of music thanatology—history, theories, and clinical narratives. *Advances, the Journal of Mind-Body Health, 9*(1), 36–48.

Turner, V. (1975). *Drama, fields, and metaphors.* New York: Cornell University Press.

Van Gennep, A. (1961). *The rites of passage.* Chicago: University of Chicago Press.

Webster's New World Dictionary. (2nd college ed.) (1982). New York: Simon & Schuster.

6 THE GRIEVING CLIENT

Grief can be mild or totally overwhelming. It is the crisis-level, overwhelming grief response that often requires nursing intervention. But the level of grief, its intrusion into one's life, can only be determined by the individual grieving and not by the particular circumstances of what provoked the grief. To help a person meet the challenges of grief, the nurse seeks to understand and enter the client's grief world.

The panorama of one overwhelming grief experience is beautifully described by a young widow:

> Grief is a tidal wave that overtakes you, smashes down upon you with unimaginable force, sweeps you up into its darkness, where you tumble and crash against unidentifiable surfaces, only to be thrown out on an unknown beach, bruised, reshaped. (Ericsson, 1993, p. 7)

Why would anyone allow themselves to value a person, relationship, or object enough to risk such pain? Because the pain of grief is "the inevitable cost of loving" (Larson & Larson, 1993,

p. 3). Healthy loving and emotional and spiritual well-being are interdependent. Those who are spiritually and emotionally healthy successfully grieve their losses by facing and feeling the pain of grief. So, love and emotional and spiritual health are intimately interwoven with grief.

GRIEF: WHAT IS IT?

Loss triggers grief. Loss triggers suffering and pain. The degree of pain experienced depends on the nature of the loss and its value to the individual. Loss of a highly valued person, relationship, or object provokes great pain. It is more than the pain of illness or injury, but also the "symptom of a spiritual wound caused by the loss" (Bozarth, 1990, p. 11). The mystery of why loss has occurred, why any loss occurs, is part of the pain of grief (Mitchell & Anderson, 1983).

   Loss also produces change, and change that cannot be stopped causes transition (Murphy, 1990). The grief work accompanying the loss must be accomplished for successful transition to occur . . . for one to incorporate the loss into one's life and perception of reality.

Grief as Crisis

Grief is a component of all our losses, however minor. Grief becomes a crisis when the loss produces a "turning point" that upsets the equilibrium, and is perceived as a "threat to self"; "when coping responses to stress fail, and the event is experienced as overwhelming" (see chapter 1 for a discussion of crisis and related references).

   Crises associated with losses are both situational and maturational (see chapter 1). As one moves through life's maturational stages, roles and relationships change, losses occur as gains are achieved. Successful grief work for each of these losses requires facing, feeling, and working through the associated pain. If the individual is unable to complete the grief work at the time of the loss, the grief will surface at the time of a future loss. Some losses associated with maturation can produce maturational crises, especially if unresolved grief work remains from former losses.

Situational crises—those posing a threat to one's steady state—are usually associated with crisis-level grief responses. Crisis-level grief requires a process of transition to incorporate the loss into reality.

What is the role of the caregiver in assisting with this successful transition? How does a holistic nurse plan care most effectively for bereaved and grieving clients? Before addressing care, a brief overview of the sources and manifestations of grief is in order.

THE GRIEF PROCESS DESCRIBED

Understanding the factors that affect grief, what processes underlie grief, and what constitutes normal and abnormal grieving can help the nurse work with the client to determine how to best mobilize resources to meet the challenges of the grief response.

For What Do We Grieve?

Attachment and separation underlie the grief response. When we invest ourselves in emotional attachments to persons and things, separation from these provokes a strong sense of loss. From the separation of birth throughout life, attachment and separation are necessary accompaniments to growth and development. Loss, however, evokes grief, so grief is an inevitable part of life.

There are numerous types of loss. Mitchell and Anderson (1983) described six major types of loss:

1. Material loss, of a physical object or of familiar surroundings

2. Relationship loss, through death, divorce, moving, job change, or change in personal friendships

3. Intrapsychic loss, or loss of an emotionally important self image, of opportunities, possibilities, or dreams

4. Functional loss, of muscular or neurological functions

5. Role loss, of social role or place in a social network

6. Systemic loss, when usual functions are no longer performed in an interdependent interpersonal system (the system as well as individuals may experience loss).

For purposes of this discussion on grief, loss of a significant person through death will serve as the example.

Variables that affect the way loss is experienced are associated with circumstances surrounding the loss, and with the way the individual has learned to deal with powerful emotions (Mitchell & Anderson, 1983, p. 51). Circumstances that affect the experience depend on whether the loss is:

1. avoidable versus unavoidable,

2. temporary versus permanent,

3. actual versus imagined,

4. anticipated versus unanticipated,

5. leaving versus being left.

For instance, an anticipated, unavoidable loss often causes a lesser degree of agony at the time of loss than an avoidable, unanticipated loss.

A person responds to the powerful emotions of crisis-level grief by using the same coping strategies as used in the past to deal with other powerful emotions. A person who is able to accept and handle such emotions will identify and acknowledge the emotions, allow the emotions to be felt, and talk through the experience. Persons who have not coped successfully with intense emotions in the past will use mechanisms such as denial, projection, withdrawal, or depression to avoid the experience, or will express intense and inappropriate anger to release the energy but avoid dealing with the other emotions experienced.

The Normal Grief Experience

Complex feelings, physical sensations, thought patterns, and behaviors are frequently expressed by bereaved persons (Worden, 1991; Mitchell & Anderson, 1983). Among these are numbness, sadness, emptiness, loneliness, isolation, yearning, fear and anxiety, guilt and shame, self-reproach, anger, sadness and despair, helplessness, hopelessness, low self-esteem, fatigue, and somatization. Fear and anxiety have been refined to include the dread of abandonment, the anxiety of separation, and fear of the future. Some individuals also express a sense of relief or emancipation, and often express discomfort with these feelings.

Commonly described physical sensations may occur, often in periodic waves of somatic distress. Frequently reported sensations include tightness in the throat or chest, hollowness in the stomach, shortness of breath, muscle weakness, dry mouth, throbbing heart, lack of energy, oversensitivity to noise, and a sense of depersonalization. Bone aching, especially limb pain, is often described. Physical symptoms include headache, insomnia, appetite loss, indigestion, bowel changes, weight loss, fatigue, and dizziness.

Thought patterns common to early grief are disbelief, denial, confusion, and difficulty concentrating. A sense of presence and preoccupation with the lost person may occur early or may persist for a time. Transient visual and auditory hallucinations are not uncommon, especially in the first weeks following the loss.

Behaviors frequently associated with normal grieving include sleep disturbances, appetite disturbances (markedly increased or decreased), absent-minded behavior, social withdrawal and loss of interest in the outside world, dreams of the deceased, avoiding reminders of the deceased or other loss, visiting places or carrying objects that remind the survivor of the deceased, treasuring objects that belonged to the deceased, searching for and calling out to the person, sighing, restless overactivity, and crying. Normal grief has many similarities to depression, and may lead to depression. Sleep disturbance, appetite disturbance, and intense sadness are classic symptoms of both grief and depression, but it is the loss of self-esteem associated with clinical depression that differentiates it from normal grief (Worden, 1991).

Body, Mind, Spirit

By 1988, serious research in psychoneuroimmunology (PNI) was providing substantial evidence for a direct brain-immune system feedback loop that may account for the higher rates of illness among people who are recently bereaved. Cowley, Brown, Howard, and Barish (1988) proposed that the evidence suggests that cells themselves experience grief or other emotions. The psychoneurological effect on the immune system puts the cells at greater than normal risk.

Stages of Grief

The grief process is often described as occurring in stages. The number of stages and what labels are applied to them varies, but the broad stages, or "generalized patterns of growth" (p. 69), identified by Manning (1984), seem useful. First, there is a period of shock. During this period, the common element is numbness. The length of this shock stage varies from days to a month or more. The numbness protects from overwhelming, unbearable pain. As the numbness ebbs, the reality stage begins. During this stage, most of the elements of agony are experienced. The reaction stage may occur simultaneously with other stages. Reactions occur sporadically and include irrational anger, guilt, hurt, frustration, fear, and helplessness. Finally, the recovery stage begins, when the individual begins to integrate the loss into the reality of life and decides to live again. Duration of the reality, reaction, and recovery stages is quite variable. The course of grief after the death of a close loved one was once thought to take about a year. Now the time frame is extended to two, maybe three years, depending on many factors surrounding the attachment and the loss itself.

Donnelley (1987) described three grief stages: shock, hurt, and healing. The shock stage differs little from that described by Manning (1984). The hurt stage has three parts, the first of which is acute pain, which may be physical as well as emotional. When the pain threatens to overwhelm, the "crazies" enter. The crazies include irrational, swiftly changing thoughts of anger, guilt, or fear, and behaviors reflecting the attempt to hold on to the person, relationship, or object that has been lost. Overwhelming reactions of anger or guilt may occur along with these crazies. When the reality of the loss is felt, a hollow ache begins. The person functions again in everyday life, but the focus is on "a deep, hollow ache and an intense inner wrestling with the phantom of meaninglessness" (p. 63). There is deep yearning and activity to keep alive the memory of what or whomever has been lost. Finally, slowly and without immediate notice, a new equilibrium begins and the person enters the stage of healing.

A cut finger—
is numb before it bleeds,
it bleeds before it hurts,
it hurts until it begins to heal,
it forms a scab and itches until
finally, the scab is gone and
a small scar is left where
once there was a wound.
Grief is the deepest wound you have
ever had. Like a cut finger,
it goes through stages and
leaves a scar. (Manning, 1984, p. 68. Used with permission.)

The Tasks of Grieving

All losses must be grieved at the time of the loss to avoid harmful emotional consequences. Suppressing the emotions of grief leads to emotional suffering and self-destructive behaviors, and "disconnects us from our internal source of self-nourishment" (Bates, 1994).

Worden (1991) determined four tasks of mourning:

1. To accept the reality of the loss

2. To work through to the pain of grief

3. To adjust to an environment in which the deceased is missing

4. To emotionally relocate the deceased and move on with life.

Accepting the reality of the loss encompasses accepting both the facts and the meaning of the loss. People seeking to protect themselves from reality may continue to deny the loss, practice selective forgetting, or deny the meaning surrounding the loss. Accepting and experiencing the pain is necessary for grief work to be concluded. People who try to avoid the pain choose to avoid feeling the whole spectrum of emotions. They use mechanisms that protect them from pain or unpleasant thoughts, such as thought stopping or substance abuse. The result of avoiding conscious grieving is often depression, requiring therapy.

Adjusting to the changed environment requires realizing all aspects of the losses involved, of all the roles played by the deceased and the role changes required by the survivor. When this task is not completed, grievers tend to promote their own helplessness.

The final task is to find an appropriate place for the deceased in the griever's emotional life that can allow him to go on living without entirely giving up the relationship with the deceased. Holding on to the past attachment leads to a resolve to never love again. Successful completion of this task brings the person to the conclusion that loving others does not mean that you love the deceased less. When all four tasks are successfully completed, the person develops a new interest in life, feels more hopeful, experiences enjoyment, and adapts to new roles.

Abnormal Grief Reactions

Abnormal grief reactions have certain characteristics that differentiate them from normal grieving. In the abnormal reaction, the individual experiences grief as overwhelming, resorts to maladaptive behaviors, and/or fails to progress through the grieving process. Worden (1991) described certain types of relationships that hinder grief and four types of complicated or dysfunctional grief reactions.

Relationships that hinder grief include highly ambivalent relationships with unexpressed hostility, those with buried wounds that reopen with the current loss, highly dependent relationships, and relationships with unresolved emotional work (the loss of "what might have been") which require grief for the lost opportunity to resolve the emotional component of the relationship along with loss of the person.

The nurse looks for abnormal grief responses in situations that put the individual at risk. Certain circumstantial and social factors make normal grieving difficult. Some of the circumstantial factors are uncertain loss, such as missing in action, or multiple losses, such as in disasters. A history of unresolved loss or complicated grief reactions predisposes a person to failure to progress through the grieving process. Social factors may affect the grief work. Normal grief is blocked by socially unacceptable losses, such as suicide, and by socially negated losses when the loss is ignored or treated as if it has not occurred. Lack of a social support network due to geography or social isolation also prevents or complicates normal grief work.

Worden (1991) described four types of complicated or dysfunctional grief reactions: chronic, delayed, exaggerated, and masked. Chronic grief reactions result in prolonged grieving that never reaches conclusion. Delayed grief reactions (also called inhibited, suppressed, or postponed) result when adequate grieving is not done at the time of the loss. The unresolved grief may be expressed at the time of a subsequent loss or of someone else's loss, and thereby appears excessive for the circumstances.

Exaggerated grief reactions result when grief is experienced as overwhelming and maladaptive behavior results. The person is aware of the loss and the maladaptive response (as opposed to masked grief reactions wherein the person is unaware of the connection between symptoms, behaviors, and the loss) (p. 73). Exaggerated reactions include major psychiatric disorders such as clinical depression, anxiety, substance abuse, post-traumatic stress disorder, or mania. Masked (or repressed) grief reactions are masked by either a physical symptom or a maladaptive behavior, but the person is unaware of the connection to grief and loss.

PLANNING CARE

Grief is an intensely individual experience, unique to each loss experienced and to each individual experiencing loss. To provide effective care, the nurse must understand the client's grief experience. The nurse must accept the client as an individual and the client's grief as a valid experience, and must convey this acceptance and a readiness to meet the client's needs. Interventions should promote self-worth and hope for the future, perceived control, and individual strengths in the face of stressors. Goals for care should be mutually set using the individual's innate drive to be healthy. If the nurse's and client's goals differ, then the nurse needs to reevaluate how well she has modeled the client's world.

Intense grief can severely deplete an individual's coping and self-care resources. The level of interruption, intrusion, or sense of encapsulation experienced by the client depends on the many factors associated with the nature of the loss and on the stage of the grieving process.

Grieving clients are often in a state of strong arousal or impoverishment during the initial stages of loss. Nursing care for a client in arousal is directed toward assisting to mobilize the client's own resources and to enhance the client's sense of control. If the client is in impoverishment, the nurse must provide any needed physical care along with psychological, emotional, and spiritual support, and should help the client begin to identify potential resources. When the client returns to a state of adaptive equilibrium, the nurse should change the focus of care to facilitate and support the client's strategies to cope.

Bates (1994) promotes an approach to grief management that supports the Modeling and Role-Modeling theory. He proposes that the caregiver's role is creative listening, mirroring what has been said, and mirroring the client's perception of reality (modeling the client's world). Bates proposes that dysfunctional grieving results from the suffering caused by suppressed emotions. The suppressed loss leads to a perception of separateness, of being vulnerable, at risk. Perception (belief) creates our reality. Therefore, suffering, as opposed to pain, is in the mind. It is a "thinking disorder." But a person cannot evaluate this harmful belief system from within oneself. The caregiver's role, then, is to discover with the client the client's ability to change his own mind. The outcome of effective grief counseling is perception adjustment. The caregiver, however, cannot adjust the client's perception. Only the clients can adjust their own perception. The caregiver's role is to create a safe "space" for dropping pretense, for healing by being genuine, open, using effective self-disclosure. Healing is a collaborative effort. Counseling skills are used not to manipulate the client, but to bring oneself into a more compassionate space.

INTERVENTIONS FOR THE STAGES OF GRIEF

In the shock stage of grief, the client is often in strong arousal. Since shock has a protective effect in the face of potentially overwhelming stress, supporting the disbelief and denial is appropriate. Assist the client to mobilize available resources, such as contacting supportive family or significant persons. Provide an environment where verbal and behavioral expressions of emotion can be openly expressed. Use creative listening and mirroring to communicate acceptance of the individual and of the expressed emotions.

If impoverishment is assessed, physical as well as psychological and emotional support may be necessary. If impoverishment continues, specialist referral may be necessary. At any point in grief management, indications of suicidal ideation should be referred to a specialist.

As shock ebbs and the reality stage begins, the client is faced with the choice to experience the pain or to escape into the "disordered thinking" involved in suffering (Bates, 1994). It is during this stage that grief management can provide the greatest assistance to help clients adjust their perceptions to perceive reality, to avoid pretense, to move through the pain.

Our culture has helped most of us, especially men, to develop behavioral skills to keep people from knowing how needy we are. Even those who are able to express their agony and talk openly of the loss are subtly pressured to stop doing so long before they should. Bates (1994) proposes that greatest healing comes to grievers through telling their story over and over and over, and over, and over, until they themselves become bored with it.

It is important to remember that clients adjust their own perceptions when they are ready to experience the pain. A nurse cannot adjust perceptions for them or manipulate them to change their mind. Mirroring the client's perception does not reinforce avoidance of reality. Rather, it reinforces a sense of being understood, of being heard, of being safe to explore alternative perceptions.

When reactions occur simultaneously with other stages, the nurse's role continues as described. Irrational anger, guilt, hurt, frustration, fear, and helplessness ebb and flow. Accepting the behaviors and expression of feelings is important. This acceptance conveys to the client a sense of being understood and of being worthy of this understanding. All efforts to encourage the client to tell the story framed in each new reaction helps move grief along. If a state of despair and impoverishment becomes evident, then referral to a specialist may be required.

When the recovery stage is reached, arousal lessens and adaptive equilibrium returns. The nurse's role becomes one of supporting the client's own coping mechanisms directed toward integrating the loss into reality and beginning to participate more fully in life and planning for the future.

The holistic nurse, who is oriented to nurturing and supporting, and able to model the client's world, encouraging this storytelling and role-model coping behaviors, is ideally suited to assisting the client through transformational grief. The nurse provides a safe space wherein the griever can see and express neediness, fear, shame—where pretense is kept at bay. The nurse's counseling skills, communication skills, and appropriate self-disclosure help to clear communication, convey understanding, reduce defenses and isolation, and encourage self-disclosure.

NURSING DIAGNOSIS

Because a normal, uncomplicated grief reaction is a normal reaction following loss, the process of nursing diagnosis associated with grief has been difficult. A grief state is a deviation from the usual life pattern, and it is associated with pain. But since normal grief reactions are normal, and the nurse's role is to facilitate the client's normal process, the authors propose that a wellness diagnosis format is most useful. The authors recommend the diagnostic wording "*opportunity to enhance* effective grieving" or "*opportunity to enhance* anticipatory grieving" (Kelley, Frisch, & Avant, 1994).

In either of the wellness grieving processes, the nurse's assessment focuses on the client's status regarding adaptive equilibrium. If maladaptive equilibrium is identified, or if factors that tend to complicate grief are assessed, then a problem-oriented or risk-oriented nursing diagnosis is generated: dysfunctional grieving or high risk for dysfunctional grieving.

Many other nursing diagnoses may become prominent in abnormal or complicated grief responses. Spiritual distress, powerlessness, hopelessness, anxiety, social isolation, ineffective individual coping, and compromised family coping are often noted when grief is complicated. Nursing care focuses on helping the client move through grief by building a trusting relationship and providing a safe space for the client to explore and experience feelings; encouraging the client to tell his story over and over; assisting the client to identify and use effective coping mechanisms; and conveying a sense of hope, love, and control.

CASE STUDY | *Stephanie*

(This case study is from Stephanie Ericsson's [1993] account of her own walk through grief. [Used with permission.] Nursing care that would have been appropriate is described.)

Stephanie was thirty-five years old and two months pregnant when her husband died. She was at the airport to meet his plane after two months of being apart when she learned of his death. Their marriage was stable but had rough patches, and was complicated by a history of infertility. Stephanie had just learned of her pregnancy when she learned of her husband's death.

At the news of his death, shock was pronounced. "The shock was . . . a big tumble into a blackness of sounds and cold hands clawing at me. Minutes were slow motion, and all that wasn't imperative to my survival was edited out of my memory" (p. 2). But shock was not completely numbing. "Every time I thought about you, I felt the slam [against a brick wall] again and again. My breath was sucked out through another opening deep inside me . . . out to oblivion" (p. 2). A bit of anger came through even early in the grief: "The doctors tried for three hours to bring you back. You refused. Oh, you were incorrigible in death as you had been in life" (p. 3). But denial was more evident: "It must be a sick joke. He's really there . . . around the next corner. As soon as I open the door, he'll be there . . . I'll catch a glimpse of him. I'm sure I do see him out of the corner of my vision, but he is never there when . . . I turn my head to catch him" (p. 8).

Reaction to others and the reactions of others to grief produce a certain social isolation at a time of greatest need for comfort. "I speak to my friends and they all have this look on their faces like they are watching me lying on the pavement with my belly sliced open . . . expression . . . of mixed pity and disgust . . . want to avert their eyes, but they can't . . . say, How are you? . . . I think, How do they think I am? . . . then one day my strength is down and I actually tell someone how I am and she can't handle it, she can't understand, and I never hear from her again" (p. 9).

The "crazies" produce irrational thoughts which increase the isolation and pain. "The accusing eyes of other people . . . their off-the-cuff remarks that scrape and cut my already skinless psyche . . . I am exposed. I am ashamed of my aloneness. Even though I know in my mind you didn't reject me, I feel that you did . . . I feel that you dumped me" (p. 13). Yet the crazies are a natural part of the grief work. Stephanie describes "a momentary lapse into sanity, where I realized that my insanity is a sane reaction to an utterly insane event" (p. 13). But "Sanity is hot, searing, and far too intense to tolerate for long. What may appear to others as crazy actions are really the appropriate way to react to the sheer powerlessness that all of us face in the shadow of death" (p. 15).

The pain is too intense, and Stephanie describes slipping into impoverishment; self-esteem slips away and depression enters. "The dreams come in the half-sleep, wet pillows, nightmares, black streaks from the mascara I wore the day I came home. I haven't worn mascara since. Why bother. For what? For whom? Don't care. Don't wash. Don't eat. Don't move. Gotta get some help. No one can help me . . . I stand on the ledge, looking over into the inevitable canyon, and what scares me the most is that I am not afraid to jump" (p. 17).

Yet within the inertia "there is something happening, like a settling of the silt after a big storm. The grains of sand have been forever rearranged. It makes no sense to do anything until all the grains have settled into their new pattern. Under the surface, the fertilizing of new life is beginning, silently, almost invisibly . . . I cannot look to tomorrow yet, for it will use up what little of today I have . . . yet deep down inside, I sense a payoff, if only I am patient" (pp. 26–27).

Finally, hope resurfaces and the recovery begins. "Loss is life's nonnegotiable side. It is the time when we learn, unconditionally, that we are powerless over things we thought we had a grip on. But it doesn't stop there, because every ending brings a new beginning . . . and I can see, in retrospect, that each one of these losses brought a blessing that would only be understood as I learned to live with the grief" (p. 29).

One final area of suppressing feelings remains for a while and is revealed in canonizing the dead. "Strange, my urge to put you into the saint category, protect you now from criticism, from the wrath of anger. As long as I think of you as a saint, I don't have to hate you for dying. I don't have to experience the emotions I would have felt about the flaws in our relationship had you lived" (p. 39).

Ultimately, Stephanie moves on through grief to emerge "different, taller, stronger, more armored, more soft" (p. 45), with fewer moments of "intolerable pain . . . anger" (p. 67), or guilt over functioning without her husband (p. 180). She finally arrives at a time of saying good-bye, of healing. "Time alone does not heal. It is the loyalty to life that heals . . . Time and distance can give perspective, but time itself must not be mistaken for a healer . . . what hurt us twenty years ago can be just as painful when another pain of the same sort strikes again. There will be no perfect time when all of the threads are cut and tied off neatly that saying good-bye will be entirely painless. But somehow, in a place deep within the heart, there will be a moment when all that we held on to, out of our longing, guilt, remorse, fear, will cease to be valuable. It will not be a happy time. But it will feel complete . . . Then we will be able to finally say, with heart felt sincerity, good-bye" (p. 184). Stephanie described her experience of this process. "I held on to you after you died. For dear life . . . I screamed into the hole you left—'You can't leave me! Not yet!' Slowly, the healing loosened my grip . . . I'm ready to let you go . . . Today I have given myself over to a new life" (p. 185).

Nursing Care for Stephanie

During Stephanie's initial shock of learning that her husband was dead, the nurse would recognize the crisis state of encapsulation and would assess Stephanie's adaptive potential. Stephanie described initial behaviors reflective of fluctuation between strong arousal and impoverishment. Appropriate nursing actions would focus on assisting Stephanie to mobilize any resources available and providing needed physical and emotional support. Encouraging telephone contact with relatives and assisting to organize a return trip home should be balanced with assisting Stephanie to meet basic needs for food and rest.

Communication during the initial shock phase should be focused on allowing Stephanie to express the rapidly changing emotions, including panic, denial, crying, withdrawal, and stunned silence. Remaining with her, communicating unconditional acceptance of her feelings and ways of expressing them, and assisting with basic needs helps to establish a trusting relationship. The nurse should avoid attempting to nudge a person out of the numbness and shock.

Once the shock phase eases and Stephanie begins to experience the reality of the loss, the holistic nurse would seek first to establish the meaning the loss has for Stephanie. As Stephanie tells her story—that she was thirty-five years old and two months pregnant after long-standing fertility problems, that her husband's death was unexpected and sudden, that she had hoped to improve a troubled relationship—the meaning of the multiple losses involved becomes clearer.

But it is only in an atmosphere of acceptance that Stephanie will expose her deepest feelings. The nurse must convey a willingness to listen, to hear, to share a portion of the pain by remaining in the interaction even when faced with the anger and agony being expressed. The nurse builds trust by modeling the worldview the client describes. At no time does the nurse try to move the client faster through the grieving process, nor convey a sense that the client's style of grieving is wrong or bad. The nurse listens and helps the client tell her story of the loss, the circumstances surrounding the loss, and her feelings about every aspect of the loss—unless or until the griever arrives at a time for avoiding communication.

During periods of social withdrawal and silence, the nurse must address the conflicting needs for human presence but also for withdrawal. This is a time for the "chicken soup" approach—the nurse brings food or comfort items, touches her or hugs her, if she seems receptive, to reassure her of the nurse's continued availability, but allows the distance.

When Stephanie's behaviors reflected reactions or the crazies, the nurse would accept the behaviors. The nurse would help Stephanie recognize that the behaviors and feelings are a normal part of the grief work. Attentive listening can provide a caring space in which the client can tell her story over and over, including the new themes as feelings ebb and flow, intensify and moderate.

As Stephanie slipped into the depression of impoverishment when the pain became too intense, the nurse would be vigilant for signs of clinical depression and suicidal ideation. Referral for specialist support may be needed. Behaviors and verbal descriptions reflecting a significant lowering of self-esteem accompanying the sleep and appetite disturbance are indicative of severe depression.

But Stephanie was able to survive this period without the specialist support, even though she herself was aware of the need for help. It is possible that she was sustained by her awareness that within the inertia something was happening to reorganize the "grains of sand" and "new life was beginning" (pp. 26–27). The nurse's role would be to help Stephanie explore her sense of inertia and her beginning awareness of a nearly imperceptible change taking place. However slight, the change could provide a basis for reestablishing hope that in the future the pain will lessen . . . that, indeed, there is a future.

Once a sense of hope resurfaces and the recovery stage begins, the nurse helps Stephanie to explore again the meaning of the losses experienced, this time relating them to the new beginning which becomes apparent. The nurse "accompanies" Stephanie through the transition of letting go of her husband, of learning to incorporate her grief into her life, of learning to take on the roles her husband is not there to carry out, and to let go of the guilt associated with being able to carry out these roles without him. The nurse accepts Stephanie's temporarily canonizing and idealizing her husband, her holding on to him. Helping Stephanie talk through her guilt and fears will help her arrive at the point of saying good-bye and choosing to go on with life.

Discussion

Key elements of grief work include recognizing that each grief experience is individual, that the time frame for progress through grief stages is individual, and that facing the pain or grief at the time the loss occurs facilitates grief work. The major focus of care is to facilitate grief work and provide physical and emotional support needed to best allow grief work to progress. The caregiver creates a safe environment or space for the client to drop pretense and openly explore and express the entire spectrum of feelings brought forth by intense grief. Through conveying a sense of presence, acceptance, and understanding of the client's grief experience, the nurse can walk with the client through the darkness and into a renewed sense of hope, as together the nurse and client discover the client's capacity to change her mind about her perception of reality.

Nursing Diagnosis	Goal	Intervention
High risk for dysfunctional grieving r/t husband's sudden death, troubled marital relationship with long-standing infertility, and recently identified two-month pregnancy	Client will progress through stages of grief, ultimately incorporating the loss into her life and choosing to accept the new life to be lived.	**Shock Stage:** 1. Assist client to meet basic needs for nutrition and rest. 2. Assist to mobilize available resources, such as calling family, friends; organizing travel home. 3. Provide human touch, hand holding, hugs, as acceptable to client. 4. Use presence and active listening to encourage client to express feelings about loss. 5. Avoid judging client's behavioral or verbal style of expressing grief; convey acceptance. **Reality and Reaction Stage:** 1. Use active listening to encourage client to explore meaning of loss and to identify all losses associated with the death. 2. Attempt to understand the client's view of the loss and reflect this understanding (model the client's world). 3. Monitor the level of adaptive potential. Assist the client to mobilize available emotional and physical resources. Refer to specialist if impoverishment results in severe depression or suicidal ideation. 4. Encourage the client to tell her story over and over again. 5. Accept periods of social isolation as normal. Provide support and communicate continued availability by bringing food or other useful items; touch or hug client if she finds this acceptable. **Recovery Stage:** 1. Use active listening and therapeutic skills to assist client to identify glimmers of hope for a future life; and to reach the conclusion of active grief work.
High risk for spiritual distress r/t sudden death of husband	Client will reestablish satisfying relationship with God and significant others; will verbalize sense of hope, meaning, and purpose in life at conclusion of active grief work.	1. Use therapeutic communication, especially active listening, to encourage the client to explore feelings of hopelessness, purposelessness, abandonment by God. Discover with the client her ability to change her mind, to change her perceptions as grief work progresses to recovery. 2. Accept client's expressions of anger toward God and others.

TABLE 6.1   *Nursing Care Plan: Stephanie*

Stephanie describes her own grief experience without noting any assistance. She describes a unique response to intense and multiple losses occasioned by her husband's sudden and untimely death. She describes how the numbness of shock protected her from overwhelming pain, but also her ability to walk into and finally through the pain. This experience may have been facilitated by her journal writing wherein she could openly and safely express all manner of feelings.

A holistic nurse's care would certainly have provided great support, especially through the period of social isolation and impoverishment. It is possible that the suffering may have been reduced by Stephanie's telling her story over and over to the nurse skilled in modeling her worldview and who was able to discover with Stephanie her own capacity for self-healing, for reformulating her reality.

SUMMARY

Accepting grief to be an intensely individual experience, unique to each loss and to each individual, is essential to providing skillful nursing care. Interventions focus on helping the client recognize available strengths and resources during different stages in the grieving process, meeting basic needs during times of impoverishment, and supporting client efforts to maintain a sense of control and hope. Assisting the client to identify the loss and experience the grief at the time of the loss can help to prevent future crises and abnormal grief responses. As the smashing, sweeping, bruising tidal wave of grief subsides, the nurse can provide support for the client's recognizing the new strength gained from surviving the grief experience and reaching the point of deciding to live life again, renewed or at least reshaped.

References

Bates, B. (1994). Life Appreciation Seminars. Aventura, FL 33180.

Bozarth, A. R. (1990). *A journey through grief.* Minneapolis, MN: Comp Care.

Cowley, G., Brown, L., Howard, J., & Barish, E. (1988, November 7). Body and soul. *Newsweek,* pp. 88–92.

Donnelley, N. (1987). *I never know what to say.* New York: Ballantine Books.

Ericsson, S. (1993). *Companion through the darkness: Inner dialogues on grief.* Glenview, IL: HarperCollins.

Kelley, J., Frisch, N., & Avant, K. (1994, April). *A trifocal model of nursing diagnosis: A wellness perspective.* Paper presented at the Eleventh Biennial Conference of the North American Nursing Diagnosis Association, Nashville, TN.

Larson, H., & Larson, I. (1993). *Suddenly single* (2nd ed.). San Francisco: Halo Books.

Manning, D. (1984). *Don't take my grief away.* San Francisco: HarperCollins.

Mitchell, K., & Anderson, S. (1983). *All our losses/all our griefs.* Belleville, MI: Spring Harbor Dist.

Murphy, S. A. (1990). Human responses to transitions: A holistic nursing perspective. *Holistic Nursing Practice, 4*(3), 1–7.

Worden, J. W. (1991). *Grief counseling and grief therapy* (2nd ed.). New York: Springer.

7 THE FAMILY UNDERGOING CHALLENGES TO HEALTH AND PEACE

To begin a discussion of families, a nurse must remember that a family—a group of persons—can be the client or recipient of care. A family can be a group of persons living together or living separately. They can be biologically related to one another, or be unrelated. They are a group of persons who have significant emotional bonds to one another. Most of the time, the nurse will meet one member of a family—the "target patient," if you will—and be called upon to help that individual deal with a life event. Often, caring interactions with a patient lead the nurse to understand that what is happening to the individual patient has significant impact on those persons close to the patient. Thus, nurses need to broaden their perspective of the client to include a group of persons.

It becomes especially clear that nurses must attend to families when a life event of one person is an unwanted crisis, a major health deviation, or a life-threatening situation. The nurse will have to assist the family to help the individual facing the challenges, while at the same time help the family members cope with their own reactions, feelings, and personal challenges.

Caring for a family is more complex than providing care to an individual. The nurse has more variables to consider, and more factors that will affect interventions and outcomes. However, considering the individual and the family, the nurse increases options for care and support, and can facilitate recovery of health and/or peace by assisting all involved to find solutions to their situations.

THE FAMILY AS A SYSTEM

It was proposed years ago that a family unit be considered a system. Systems theory proposes that the unit (family) is made up of individuals who are emotionally connected, such that any event that impacts one member will impact the others as well. By way of example, consider the impact on a four-person family (mother, father, boy child, and girl child) when the following events occur:

- The birth of a baby
- A significant promotion at work for the mother
- The father facing a diagnosis of cancer
- The boy having significant school difficulties
- The girl leaving home for college

It is clear that each of these events significantly affects each of the family members. Some of the events are positive, happy, maturational events; others are problems with an emotionally negative impact. Nonetheless, each event creates an adjustment for the family.

Systems theory states that when people (or things) are connected in some meaningful way, events that affect one part of the system will necessitate an adjustment in all other parts of the system. It is helpful to think of a family as in balance. A family works to achieve a state of equilibrium. Then something happens to one member. The equilibrium is upset, and the relationships, supports, and tasks of everyday living need to be readjusted. This is exactly what happens to families seen by nurses. One member of the family is the "target patient" — the person who is seeking nursing care. All other members of the family are reacting, readjusting, and making every effort to establish a new equilibrium. Keeping in mind the meaning of the family as a system, and accepting that the unit of care is the family group, the nurse has many tools for assessing and evaluating a family, and making plans for interventions.

FAMILY ASSESSMENT

Duvall's Theory of Family Development

Many frameworks have been suggested for family assessment. The authors believe that the concept of family development is useful and consistent with the Modeling and Role-Modeling theory presented throughout this book. The developmental model taught widely to nurses is the framework of Evelyn Duvall (1977)—describing families in developmental stages as they grow, mature, and move along the life span. First, Duvall presents family tasks; that is, general tasks that a family is expected to accomplish for its members (physical maintenance, allocation of resources, division of labor, socialization of members, reproduction, maintenance of order, and placement of members into society). These are tasks that make sense when one considers the roles families have in society. These family tasks provide one means of assessing family functioning. For example, if a family is accomplishing these tasks, it could be considered to be functioning well; if it is not accomplishing most of these tasks, it could be considered dysfunctional.

The major framework of Duvall's theory, however, is the concept of family development. She states that families pass through developmental stages in a similar way as an individual passes through developmental stages. Duvall's developmental stages are based on the assumption of a married couple living as a nuclear family, having children, and defining themselves and their development as a family in relation to the age and developmental stages of their children (see table 7.1). This model, while helpful for some situations, is no longer useful for the

Stage 1:	Beginning families; new marriage partners
Stage 2:	Childbearing; families with infants
Stage 3:	Families with preschool children
Stage 4:	Families with school-age children
Stage 5:	Families with teenage children
Stage 6:	Families with young adult children
Stage 7:	Families with adult children
Stage 8:	Aging Families

TABLE 7.1   *Stages of Family Development According to Duvall*

majority of families a nurse encounters. How often do nurses see a family as a unit where a couple marries in their young adulthood, has children, and remains as an intact unit until the children grow up and leave home, with the parents left as "aging family members" (Duvall's final stage)? A nurse using Duvall's framework quickly sees that modern American families are often in several of Duvall's stages at once. For example, the married couple may be a new couple beginning a married relationship (stage 1) who are also raising teenagers (stage 5), becoming childbearing (stage 2), and supporting aging parents (stage 7).

Duvall's framework provides nurses with a way to assess how truly complicated modern family life is, but it does not provide much direction in planning care and support for families. The authors have found that another theory, another way of looking at families, is more helpful in practice. That theory is Bowen's (1970) model of describing family development in a different way.

Bowen's Family Systems Theory

Bowen began with a biological model, viewing persons as having both an emotional and an intellectual level of functioning. The emotional level is associated with lower brain centers and relates to feelings. The intellectual level is associated with the cerebral cortex or higher brain centers and relates to cognition. Bowen suggests that the emotional and intellectual systems of an individual are connected neurologically, and that the degree of connectedness varies among persons. This degree of connectedness between the emotional and intellectual systems of a person dramatically affects the person's functioning. To be fully functional, particularly in such social situations as a family group, an individual should have a balance between the thinking and feeling components. Indeed, observations of families have shown that many dysfunctional families are unable to distinguish between the intellectual process of thinking and the subjective process of feeling.

To further describe the balance of the emotional and intellectual systems, Bowen describes an individual's growth over time as *differentiation*. Differentiation is, of course, a biological term that involves the development of a cell, wherein the cell becomes set apart as a specific kind of cell; for example, a nerve cell, a muscle cell, or a skin cell. Differentiation means that the cell is mature, no longer a unit that has not yet developed. It is useful to think about the process of differentiation as that of unfolding, growth, and maturation.

When applying this term to human development, Bowen describes the balance between the emotional and intellectual components of a person. A low level of differentiation means that there is little connection between a person's emotions and intellect. A high level means that there is a strong connection. At least theoretically, there is a continuum with no level of differentiation (connectedness) at one end, and a high level of differentiation at the other. It is useful to think about differentiation as existing in low, moderate, and high levels. These levels are best described in terms of both child and adult behaviors.

Low Level of Differentiation   A person with a low level of differentiation is governed by emotions. This person lives in the present and has an instinctual worldview. Feelings and repetitive behaviors dominate. Because feelings are so prominent, the person experiences a relatively high degree of anxiety. The person who lives in the present is unable to think ahead or behave in a goal-directed manner. Many of the person's actions are impulsive.

A two-year-old child readily exhibits behaviors and actions consistent with a low level of differentiation. The child lives in the present, knows what he wants, and cannot understand the concept of "delayed gratification." The child wants what he wants now! Emotions dominate actions. The child laughs or cries, experiences fear and anger, love and hate, all within a few moments. Intimate interpersonal relationships are not possible, because the child cannot give empathy, understanding, or love to another. The child at this age is only able to accept and enjoy the attentions of another.

Young children are not the only individuals who exhibit low levels of differentiation. There are many adults who have not developed the connections between their emotional and intellectual components. These adults may be functioning well in other aspects of their lives—for example, they may be fully employed and successful in work roles. However, their emotions dominate relationships with others, such that they are unable to form intimate relationships. They make decisions impulsively and based on emotions. Intense, short-term, often serial relationships are common. The adult functioning at this level is not able to step back from a situation and analyze what is happening, and instead reacts emotionally to situations. With these patterns, conflicts can readily escalate into violence.

Moderate Level of Differentiation   A person at this stage of development is less dominated by the emotional system. However, emotions dominate much of the person's relationships. Intellectually, the person tends to engage in dualistic thinking. The person views the world in terms of black and white. Things are either good or bad; people are either smart or stupid, loved or rejected. The person may have a closeness to another, but finds that in a positive relationship he will "fuse" or enmesh with the other person. The goal of relationships is to please the other person, and the individual loses himself.

People at this level form relationships, some of which last over periods of years. However, these people find that life becomes rule bound. They do "what is right" and stick to rules, commitments, and decisions. They expect others to do the same and they are judgmental. Such an individual is unable to see the context of a situation or comprehend that an understanding of the context of a situation could lead to a different understanding of the event. A person at a moderate level of differentiation is unable to "step into another person's shoes," and cannot see the world from another's perspective.

High Level of Differentiation   People at a high level of differentiation have a better balance of emotions and intellect. These people express emotions and understand them at the same time. They are able to feel anger and step back from that anger to understand what caused it. These people are able to temper anger by using intellectual functioning. They exhibit relativistic thinking and are able to understand the contextual nature of the world. Decisions are not a matter of rules or a matter of doing what is right or doing what is expected. Rather, decisions are made on the basis of the context, the impact, and the outcome. A person at this level of differentiation can form intimate relationships and appreciate the uniqueness of self and of others.

Family Dynamics and Level of Differentiation

Families take on a character that reflects the level of differentiation of the adult family members. Families whose adult members operate at a low level of differentiation exhibit impulsive patterns of interactions. They make decisions without thinking through the effects and consequences. They relate on an emotional level. They often exhibit spousal abuse and other forms of domestic violence, as they are unable to use intellectual powers to check an emotion as strong as anger.

A family whose adult members have developed to a moderate level of differentiation exhibits rigid patterns of interactions. The family is bound by rules and order. Each family member is expected to have defined roles and the family does not tolerate any variations in expected roles or behaviors.

In contrast, a family whose adult members have developed to a high level of differentiation is flexible in its interactions. The family actively seeks to support all of its members. Because the adults are able to see the world from another person's perspective, the family understands each member as unique and encourages family members to develop differently from one another. Family roles are ascribed on the basis of knowledge, skill, and interest. Table 7.2 presents a summary of family patterns according to level of differentiation.

Differentiation:	Low	Moderate	High
Mode of Operation	Emotions dominate relationships	Emotions dominate relationships/intellect plays a role	Emotions and intellect in balance
Anxiety Level	High	Moderate	Low
Thought Patterns	Live in present/will not think ahead	Dualistic thinking	Relativistic thinking
Family Dynamics	Impulsive	Rigid	Flexible

TABLE 7.2   Level of Differentiation and Family Patterns

Nursing Actions Based on Family Differentiation

Nurses must understand the underlying family dynamics in order to model the family's world and facilitate healthy interactions. Assessment of the family level of differentiation is the single most important aspect of understanding family dynamics. If a nurse knows the family's level of differentiation, the nurse also knows how the family thinks, what is important to the family, and how to communicate with the family on an appropriate level. Some examples follow.

Knowing that a family is at a low level of differentiation, a nurse will seek to develop trust with the family and provide experiences that will help the adults develop cognitive skills to understand their emotions. The literature provides examples of how nurses and therapists help impulsive, violent persons deal with anger, and these are excellent examples of effective ways of dealing with persons with low differentiation. One technique includes having a person keep an "anger journal," wherein the client keeps track of when the anger occurred and what brought it on. The person is taught to identify the anger and accept it as part of living. Further, the person is asked to remove herself from the situation so that escalation of the emotion cannot occur. Drinking and driving must be avoided. The person learns to take time out by going for a walk or engaging in some other non-hurtful activity until the anger cools down. Thus, the person learns in the instance of anger, how intellectual skills—that is, identifying the anger and using a contract to perform some non-hurtful activity—can be used to avoid negative expressions of the emotion. In this process, the person learns one method of using intellectual functioning to balance an emotion. For many people this is the first step in moving toward a higher level of differentiation.

Working with a family at a moderate level of differentiation, the nurse knows that the family operates through rules and expectations. Sometimes the rules work well for most of the family members, but not well for all of them. For example, a family may have an expectation that all family members play sports. Any persons in such a family who are not athletically inclined may be made to feel as if they are no good. A nurse can focus interventions on assisting the family to see that each member is unique, and that all may not live up to the same standards. Any intervention that can help the family develop flexibility and understanding of both their similarities and differences can help this family move to a higher level. Families at a moderate level of differentiation can predictably have trouble adjusting when a family member becomes ill and unable to perform assigned roles. In these families, persons need assistance in finding support and resources in carrying out family tasks when the order they require disintegrates.

The family at a high level of differentiation needs nursing care that facilitates members' own abilities to feel emotions and understand events. The family members have many skills in dealing with their own situations, but will often seek nursing care at a time of crisis. They need information from the nurse, help with understanding it, and someone with whom to talk about events and options.

Nurses often approach all families as if they were at a high level of differentiation, despite the fact that most of the families a nurse sees are operating at a lower level. Perhaps this is the reason nurses are so often frustrated that families do not listen, or call families "problem cases" or "noncompliant." Careful assessment permits a nurse to plan interactions at each family's level, and leads to effective communication and interventions.

MODELING AND ROLE-MODELING AND THE FAMILY UNIT

The Adaptive Potential Assessment Model (APAM) (Erickson, Tomlin, & Swain, 1983) can be applied to families as well as to individuals. The APAM is another means of assessment that helps a nurse decide when to attempt interventions and when to wait. The APAM framework invites us to think of a family as being in adaptive equilibrium, maladaptive equilibrium, arousal, or impoverishment. Experienced nurses have seen families in all these conditions, although without words to describe the condition, one cannot fully use one's observations in practice.

A family in equilibrium functions in an established pattern and has no incentive for change. The family's equilibrium may be adaptive or maladaptive. Adaptive equilibrium is a condition where the needs of all family members are being met, the family tasks are being accomplished, and each family member feels valued, loved, and supported by the other family members. A family in maladaptive equilibrium also functions in an established pattern. However, the needs of all members are not being met. At least one member of the family is being used to meet the needs of someone else. A family member is feeling ridiculed, left out, or unsupported. Until the situation reaches a crisis, there is little incentive for change. The crisis could be anything that upsets the balance, for example, a suicide, a jail term, a child failing in school, or one family member's expression of intolerance for the situation. When the equilibrium is upset, the family moves to arousal.

Just as with an individual in arousal, a family in arousal experiences anxiety over a specific event. That event may be an illness, a financial crisis, a move, or a family fight. Because the family's equilibrium is upset, the family must accommodate and reestablish equilibrium. The family mobilizes resources, and the nurse must help the family to identify and mobilize the resources they have. Family members in arousal will express emotions, and should be helped to understand the feelings that their situation brings on. Members of a family in arousal may be willing to look at their own family dynamics and begin to understand why their equilibrium state was maladaptive. A family in arousal is motivated to change, whereas a family in equilibrium is not.

A family in impoverishment has no energy, no hope, and no sense of resources. Such a family needs nursing and social services to provide a secure and stable environment from which to build again an equilibrium that allows the family to see a future. A nursing role is to identify that the impoverishment exists and to understand that this family needs direct care and is unable to "rise to the occasion." The nurse (and the health care system) should avoid making demands on this family that the family has no means to meet.

THE FAMILY AND NURSING DIAGNOSIS

Three nursing diagnoses that identify the family as the client are approved by the North American Nursing Diagnosis Association (NANDA). These are alteration in family process, ineffective family coping, and impaired home maintenance management. Using these diagnoses helps the nurse identify that it is the family group needing nursing care.

Carpenito (1993) distinguishes between alteration in family process and ineffective family coping as follows. Altered family process is used for a usually supportive family that is experiencing a stressor that challenges its previously effective functioning. Ineffective family coping is used for a family that is not usually supportive, but is destructive in its ability to manage internal or external stressors. Thus, a family in arousal because of a terminal illness of a family member exhibits altered family processes; a family that exhibits any degree of domestic violence that is coping with a crisis such as the teenager who has run away can be diagnosed as ineffective family coping. It is not the situation but rather the family's ability to function, to cope, and/or to react to the situation that determines the correct diagnostic label.

The last diagnosis that addresses the family unit is impaired home maintenance management. This diagnosis is used for the family that is unable to maintain a safe, hygienic, growth-producing home environment. Impaired home maintenance management should be used as a diagnosis when the family exhibits difficulty in maintaining the home environment over time, not merely in response to an identified crisis. The etiology for impaired home maintenance management could be lack of knowledge, finances, mobility, and/or access to services.

CASE STUDY | *The Johnson Family*

Emily, a 29-year-old woman, visits the public health nurse this morning at a women's safe house. Emily has been married for seven years and has three daughters—Maria (6 years), Susan (4 years), and Betty (1½ years). Emily came to the safe house last night after she and her husband had a fight. Her husband, Joe (age 32) hit her several times with his fists and left the house. He had threatened to strike the children, so Emily sought help and refuge at the safe house.

Emily's marriage has been speckled with abusive incidents for the past five years. She and Joe get into fights easily when something happens to create tension within the home—the girls getting sick, the dinner not being ready on time, the telephone ringing too often, the washing machine breaking. Emily had a job as a clerk in a department store, but she had to quit shortly before Betty was born due to demands of the pregnancy and the child care demands of the other girls. Joe works as a carpenter and has had reasonably steady employment until very recently. They have had financial difficulties since then, and there never seems to be quite enough money to cover rent, food, and clothing.

Emily relates that the family rarely eats a meal together in the home—they always have their television on, and the girls watch television anytime they want. Meals are eaten in the living room. Joe leaves for work early in the morning, before the children are up, and returns home after the workday. He spends much of his free time with his friends. They hang out down the street, doing nothing in particular. When Joe is out of work, he spends much of his time watching television, reading the paper, and meeting his friends. Over the past two years, he has increased his alcohol consumption and Emily thinks he "drinks too much" two or three times per week.

They engage in some family outings (a walk on the beach, a trip to the zoo). Emily states that these outings occur when things are going well for the family. Right now, Emily is physically tired and feeling emotionally drained. She says she feels helpless. The girls have slept well in the safe house and are playing with other children. They do not seem bothered by the impending family crisis. Emily states, "I know I have to change this marriage or leave it. I've had enough and now is the time to get help." Emily is sure that Joe will be very angry that she has left. Emily left once about six months ago and went to her sister's house. That time, Joe came right over and told her to go home. He said then, as he has said many times before, that he does not mean to harm her or the children, he just acts before he knows what has happened.

The nurse, Mary Anne, assesses that the family is at a low level of differentiation. Their family dynamics have been impulsive—they are unable to talk to each other, they have little, if any, real person-to-person interaction. Emily's leaving home to come to a safe house will put the family into a state of arousal—this family is now facing a crisis. However, individually, Emily is in a state of impoverishment this morning. The nurse recognizes that the family must deal with the following:

1. A confrontation of the spousal abuse

2. Joe's state of anger, and his history of not being able to deal with anger

3. Emily's feelings of helplessness

There are three priority nursing diagnoses that Mary Anne will use to plan her care with the family. The first is a family nursing diagnosis—ineffective family coping r/t history of domestic violence, and inability to react to unexpected events of living without anger. The second diagnosis relates to Emily—hopelessness r/t feeling trapped in an abusive relationship and r/t her current state of impoverishment. The third diagnosis addresses Joe—potential for violence r/t inability to handle feelings of anger.

Mary Anne first addresses Emily. Because she is in a state of impoverishment, Emily needs direct care. Mary Anne believes that Emily knows what she needs, and if asked, will tell her. Emily responds that she needs rest and wants to take a nap. Mary Anne fixes Emily a snack of tea and toast, and arranges for the safe house staff to care for the children while Emily sleeps this morning. Emily says she needs to call her husband, but she will do so later.

Mary Anne also recognizes that in spite of being in impoverishment this morning, Emily was in arousal last night. Last night, Emily took her daughters and left home; she mobilized resources available to her by coming to the safe house. Emily needs direct care this morning, but the nurse expects that soon Emily will move back into arousal as she deals with her marriage and her future. Emily will need the support of the staff to continue mobilizing resources and to reestablish equilibrium.

Mary Anne's plan for work with the family includes: assisting Emily with direct care and physical safety over the next several days; supporting Emily to call Joe, and requesting that Joe meet with a counselor regarding his abusive behaviors, promoting an establishment of family communications; and assisting the family to mobilize resources that will help them establish a new equilibrium.

In carrying out these plans, Mary Anne found that Emily and Joe decided to live apart for a while, that Emily and the children established themselves in a new state of equilibrium, and that Emily and Joe used resources in their community to seek counseling that could help them to establish a different, more supportive relationship. This family had work that was ongoing; the nurse used a theory perspective to help them understand what resources they needed and encouraged them to begin a path toward a healthier relationship.

Discussion

In this case study, the nurse uses family theory to assess the family dynamics and relationships. Further, she uses the language of nursing diagnoses to identify those concerns for which professional nursing has a role. The nurse addresses both family and individual problems in order to best facilitate health and growth for the family as a whole. Viewing the family as the client moves nursing care and interventions to a different level of complexity, as both the individuals' and the family's needs are taken into account.

SUMMARY

Nurses are often called upon to assist a family, as a client group, to meet the difficult challenges they face. Viewing the family as a system—that is, understanding that any event or situation affecting one family member will have an impact on the others—helps the nurse to understand and interpret behaviors of individuals. Family theory, particularly the work of Duvall and Bowen, provides a grounding for assessment and evaluation. Family nursing diagnoses identified by NANDA offer a cogent language for nurses to communicate family concerns to one another and provide a firm basis for planning and evaluating nursing care. Nurses' work with families becomes a major concern in any effort to assist individuals to find peace and health.

References

Bowen, M. (1978). *Family therapy in clinical practice*. New York: Jason Aronson.

Carpenito, L.J. (1993). *Nursing diagnosis: Application to clinical practice* (5th ed.). Philadelphia: J.B. Lippincott.

Duvall, E.R. (1977). *Marriage and family development*. Philadelphia: J.B. Lippincott.

Erickson, H., Tomlin, E., & Swain, M.A. (1983). *Modeling and Role-Modeling: A theory and paradigm for nursing*. Lexington, SC: Pine Press.

Shealy, A.H. (1988). Family therapy. In C. Beck, R. Rawlins, & S. Williams (Eds.), *Mental health psychiatric nursing: A holistic life-cycle approach* (pp. 543–558). St. Louis: C.V. Mosby.

4

TOOLS FOR AVOIDING CRISES

8 NURSES AND ORGANIZATIONS

A nurse may be called upon to treat an organization as a client, just as a nurse may provide care to a family group. Further, most nurses work in an organization and can feel either powerful or powerless in their jobs, depending on both the organizational style and the nurse's knowledge of how organizations work. An organization includes a collection of people who come together to work toward some end—to provide goods and/or services, or to accomplish some task. Organizations with which nurses are involved can be for-profit businesses, nonprofit service groups, governmental agencies, educational institutions, and a wide array of health care agencies.

As nurses, each of us has worked in organizations; many have firsthand knowledge of how varied organizations can be with regard to their styles or personalities. We understand that each organization has qualities that make it distinct and different from other groups. Sometimes, it even feels as though the organization has a personality of its own that is greater than that of the people within it. There are some organizations that have a crisis du jour, always dealing with some problem and never getting ahead to plan and organize activities. Others function well and seem both well-managed and well-staffed.

Like a family, an organization is made up of individual people. These people do not necessarily choose to be together; they come together for reasons of employment, skills, and interest to form a work group. They often find themselves together daily, and they need each other to accomplish their work goals. They establish patterns of interactions that depend upon the levels of maturity, honesty, and integrity of each person. Their style of interaction is based on these individual characteristics as well as the patterns of the leadership of the organization.

The authors believe that the same theories that help us to understand families can be useful in understanding organizations. For example, the level of differentiation of the organizational leadership may impact the dynamics of the entire group (see chapter 7). However, the approach taken in this chapter is how the Modeling and Role-Modeling theory can be used to understand and intervene in organizations.

ORGANIZATION ASSESSMENT

Some organizations seem to have a winning team, a group that accomplishes goals, gets along well, and works efficiently. Other organizations are just the opposite—persons do not get along and at least some individuals feel disempowered. From a different perspective, some organizations seem goal directed and run smoothly; others seem to be in a constant state of crisis. What is the difference? What can a worker or a manager do to move a group from one to the other?

First, one should assess the organization from within the Adaptive Potential Assessment Model (APAM) (Erickson, Tomlin, & Swain, 1983). First ask, "Is the organization in equilibrium, arousal, or impoverishment?" The answer will provide an important understanding of the group and will suggest interventions that may lead the group to be more efficient and productive.

An Organization in Equilibrium

An organization in equilibrium is functioning in a pattern that works or has worked for some time. The organization has a character based on its patterns—it is formal or informal, friendly or reserved, a group of team players or individualists. Like an individual in equilibrium, the organization has no incentive to change. One may hear comments such as "That's not how we do things here" or "We've always done it this way" when working in an organization in equilibrium.

The nurse must remember that equilibrium can be either adaptive or maladaptive. Like a family in adaptive equilibrium, an organization in adaptive equilibrium meets its goals and tasks. It understands that persons within the organization are unique and respects each person as able to make a contribution to the whole. Further, an organization in adaptive equilibrium promotes the professional growth and development of each person. Characteristics of an organization in adaptive equilibrium include: the organization has a clear sense of its objectives and goals; there is a feeling among its workers that the workplace is a positive environment; and the workers feel that they are part of a group. Also, the organization is flexible and able to adapt to change.

In contrast, an organization in maladaptive equilibrium is often "off track," that is, it does not meet its goals, or if it does, it does so inefficiently. There may be no consensus as to what the goals and objectives of the group are. Some may see the organization as existing for the workers; others see it as existing to provide service or to produce a product. The workers may be viewed as all being the same and may not be valued for their thoughts or ideas. The workers' needs for professional growth and development may be disregarded; or the workers may not have any interest in developing themselves. Characteristics of an organization in maladaptive equilibrium are subversive or passive-aggressive responses to change; backbiting and gossiping, which alienate people from one another; and an inflexible attitude toward change or innovation.

An Organization in Arousal

Organizations are most often in arousal when outside forces cause a disruption in their ongoing patterns. These outside forces vary. One example is the separation or resignation of a key organizational person, which forces the group to deal with a new individual hired to replace the person who left. In health care agencies, accrediting bodies are often the outside force that pushes the organization into arousal. In these situations, the accrediting bodies set standards that the persons within the agency must meet in order for the agency to remain a viable group. Meeting such accrediting criteria forces agencies' employees to work together and come to terms with the parts of the organization that do not meet the national standards. Other outside forces in health care, such as any malpractice litigation or changes in laws and/or policies regarding practice and reimbursement, can move any organization into arousal.

An organization in arousal uses whatever skills it has acquired in its past to adapt to change. The most successful organizations can be flexible and use their employees to help adapt to changes. Clearly, a group in adaptive equilibrium has a better chance to resolve external problems quickly, because a group in adaptive equilibrium has people who can work together, value each other, and create change. On the other hand, a group in maladaptive equilibrium may need the arousal to force a change. Arousal is needed to change the long-standing patterns and move the group from maladaptive to adaptive equilibrium. Managers know that this kind of arousal can be caused by a change in staffing, and this is often a good plan for moving forward a group in maladaptive equilibrium.

An Organization in Impoverishment

An organization is in impoverishment when its workers have given up on the organization. Workers (and sometimes the manager) see the organization as a more or less hopeless enterprise. An organization or unit can be thrown into impoverishment when someone decides to eliminate the unit. In these situations, the workers are looking for employment elsewhere, and there cannot be a cohesion among the group. An organization can move into impoverishment if it has been in arousal and is unable to meet the challenges required to reestablish equilibrium. If managers wish to restore a group in impoverishment, direct planning for the future of the unit and/or its employees will be necessary.

NURSES IN ORGANIZATIONS

Nurses most often work within health care organizations and can assess their own workplace, whether it is a unit within a hospital, a home health agency, or another unit. Knowing the level of adaptation of a unit helps in understanding why the organization works the way it does and provides the nurse with tools for initiating change.

The authors provide these basic recommendations for dealing with one's own work organization:

1. Evaluate your own work setting.

2. If it is in adaptive equilibrium, support those who keep it that way and value each person for his or her unique contribution to the whole.

3. If it is in maladaptive equilibrium, attempt to motivate for change. Do not involve yourself in the backbiting and gossiping that serve to separate people. Value each person for his or her contributions. Provide a positive example of flexibility and honesty to the group.

4. If the organization is in arousal, recognize this as a time for change. Align yourself with those who are working for positive change. Help the group in any way you can to reestablish an adaptive equilibrium.

5. If the organization is in impoverishment, help yourself and others to mobilize resources to understand the positive nature of the group. Get outside help; this is a time when support and caring are needed most.

The following case study is presented as an example of how this framework can be used to help nurses achieve change in their workplace.

CASE STUDY | *3-North*

Three-North (3-N) is a medical-surgical unit at Elsewhere Community Hospital. The patients in the unit are acutely ill individuals, many of whom have acute surgical conditions on top of long-term medical problems. Nurses on 3-N work eight-hour shifts and are typically assigned to work one of the three shifts.

There is a nurse manager, Shandra, and a shift supervisor for each shift—Helen (day shift), Rosa (evening shift), and Camellia (night shift). There are twelve other registered nurses on the unit, four practical nurses, eight nursing assistants, and one ward clerk.

Nursing care is provided under the primary care model, with every patient on the unit being assigned to a registered nurse. Care is documented through the nursing process. Care plans and assessments are written in standardized form and adapted to individual patients. RNs are responsibile for updating care plans each shift.

During the past five years, the staff morale at 3-N has been declining. The nurses on the evening shift believe that the nurses on the day shift purposefully leave all the paperwork for them to do. Nurses on the night shift believe that the evening shift nurses are inattentive to the needs of families. Day shift nurses are busy dealing with treatments, physician rounds, surgical schedules, nursing students, and the like, and they feel that no one really understands how hard they work.

Each shift has one or two people who carefully construct their workday so as not to be available to others who need help. It is not that these nurses do not do their job, they are just conveniently not available to do anything more than what is required. Those who do support one another recognize over time that they work harder for the same level of pay and recognition that the others receive. There are two nurses on 3-N who call in sick frequently—at least one or two days each month. These persons are in relatively poor health; however, other nurses wonder if they don't call in sick on days that are predicted to be particularly busy or difficult.

The hospital functions under a shared-governance model. However, this model has been more successful on other units than it has been on 3-N. Nurses do have governance councils, and they sit on hospital committees as part of their regular work assignments. The 3-N staff, however, does not contribute to these committees and often presents a sarcastic manner toward anyone else who is trying something new.

Shandra is a new manager to this unit who was being hired to help prepare this unit for significant changes. The hospital is to undergo a major accreditation inspection in two years. Further, the hospital plans to drastically reduce the number of surgical inpatients and fully expects the number of patients on 3-N to decrease. It is projected that within three years the 3-N staff will work both as inpatient nurses and home health nurses, in keeping with the movement of patients into the home setting. The hospital administration has considered the possibility of closing the unit and admitting all medical-surgical patients to another floor.

Shandra recognizes that the unit is in maladaptive equilibrium. There is no motivation to change, but things are not working well. With this in mind, Shandra plans to use the upcoming accreditation and the move to home health care as motivators for change. She fully expects that the change to home health care will throw the unit into arousal and sees this upheaval as good. It is not a crisis, rather it is a challenge with an opportunity to provide positive change and new direction.

While there are no nursing diagnoses that address organizations, Shandra considers the unit to be experiencing ineffective coping and ineffective work patterns. Her plan follows:

1. Ensure that all nurses recognize that successful reaccreditation is necessary for the continuance of the unit.

2. Request nurses who are most interested in home care to identify themselves and begin cross-training as home care nurses.

3. The necessary staffing changes will permit a change in coworkers for all of the nurses on 3-N.

Shandra needs to build trust, first by approaching people honestly and demonstrating that she is a capable, caring nurse. Second, Shandra will use her position to promote a positive orientation by framing the unit's changes into challenges. Shandra will help the nurses to see a future that might not be identical to their present, but one that will nonetheless be stable and satisfying work for them. And lastly, Shandra will welcome new staff and a change of staff each shift as an opportunity to alter the dynamics of interaction.

Above all, Shandra will recognize the value and contribution that each nurse makes. She will assist those who are frequently ill to identify work schedules that meet their physical needs. And she will make every effort to direct 3-N through arousal toward a new equilibrium, more adaptive than the last.

Discussion

Through the use of the Modeling and Role-Modeling theory, a nurse manager was able to assess the functioning of a hospital unit. The APAM model proved a most useful tool in understanding the group behavior and in implementing a plan of action. It becomes clear that organizations, as well as individuals, face challenges to their operations. The same tools used for working with individuals can be adapted to facilitate work with organizational groups.

SUMMARY

Nurse managers are called upon to facilitate optimal functioning of groups in their daily work. Organizations must be understood as a collection of people, with both an individual and a collective personality. Nursing theory, particularly the adaptive potential model, is used as an illustration of how nurse managers may assess and intervene with difficult situations. Nurse managers can use these theories to assess, plan, and evaluate their ability to facilitate positive change. It becomes clear that an organization may need to go through a period of arousal and upheaval in order to achieve the balance and harmony that adaptive equilibrium provides.

Reference

Erickson, H., Tomlin, E., & Swain, M.A. (1983). *Modeling and Role-Modeling: A theory and paradigm for nursing.* Lexington, SC: Pine Press.

9 | DEALING WITH CONFLICT

Evan Ferber, MA, ABS, CMHC

Just as people are greater than the sum of their components, so too, human beings are born into, nurtured, and live within human systems that are greater than their constituent parts. First each person experiences the family, and then with growth and development, the neighborhood, the local community, and so on until ultimately and ideally, the entire world community is embraced. Most of us never evolve our consciousness to be able to embrace this universal whole, but environmentally, politically, socially, and economically, our species is dimly starting to realize that each of us living on the planet at any given time is indeed but one small component of the greater whole.

The discussion in this chapter assumes that conflict is neither good nor bad. It is a primal fact of existence for human beings as social animals. What we choose to do with conflict and what our resources are for handling conflict cause it to be either a positive tool for change and healing, or a major contributor to sickness and dysfunction.

As persons move through life facing their inevitable losses, developmental tasks, and life crises, conflict is always and everywhere with them. The nurse needs a theoretical and practical grounding in conflict resolution in order to assist clients to navigate through the sea of conflict that life presents at every stage of human development.

EXPERIENCING CONFLICT FROM THE INSIDE OUT

We probably all have felt the pain of being misunderstood, discounted, verbally and/or physically abused. We have all had the two-sided primal urge to inflict pain on our opponent or run away. Deeply imbedded in our primate inheritance is this so-called "fight or flight" response. The physiological state of readiness that this response to perceived danger elicits in our bodies is also well understood. The anger arousal cycle is part of the nervous system response. Figure 9.1 illustrates the anger arousal cycle. When physiological stasis has been upset by the triggering

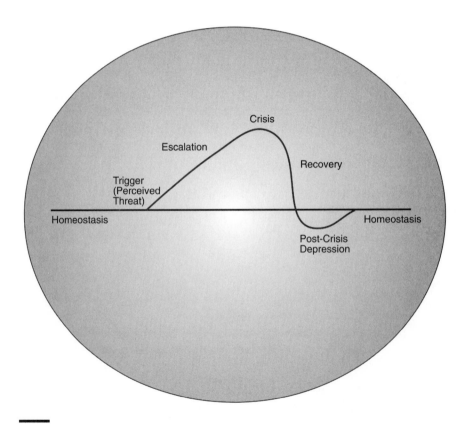

FIGURE 9.1   The anger arousal cycle.

of the alarm reaction and the adrenal system responds, the blood goes to the extremities in readiness for fight or flight. Higher cerebral functioning is limited and strong emotion in some mixture of fear and rage is experienced. The recovery phase is noteworthy in that a natural physiological depression is experienced before stasis is reestablished. Feelings of regret, loss, confusion, and sadness are common at this stage of the cycle. Whenever a person relives the event through retelling or through having to deal with the other party or parties to the conflict, the anger arousal cycle is restimulated to some degree.

DISPUTE RESOLUTION IN TRADITIONAL CULTURES

All societies have developed ways of managing the anger arousal cycle and the conflict between community members so that bloodshed is kept to within reasonable limits. All aboriginal peoples and historic high cultures have evolved processes that define the rules to be followed and the roles to be assumed by the disputants and the mediators. Often, village elders take on the mediator role. The individuals in dispute are imbedded in complex familial relationships, so most traditional dispute resolution occurs within the context of families, clans, and villages.

ALTERNATIVE DISPUTE RESOLUTION

There have been some precedents of third party mediation of interpersonal and communal conflict in European-settled North America. John Wesley taught his Methodist followers to speak their minds and negotiate their differences in regularly held group meetings. The followers of George Fox did likewise and to this day Quaker meetings practice a form of consensual decision making that requires that agreement is reached by all members on a divisive subject. In general, clergy members have been sought out to attempt mediation of family and marital conflict. However, there has not been a flourishing and pervasive tradition of dispute resolution in mainstream North American culture.

Four sources from the early 1970s have helped the spread of alternative dispute resolution (ADR) in the ensuing 15 years:

1. The Berger Court encouraged the use of nonlitigated methods of settling lawsuits as a means of keeping court dockets unclogged.

2. Three pilot community-based mediation services were funded by Griffin Bell when he was Attorney General under president Jimmy Carter. (The Atlanta Justice Center is still a seminal institution in the field.)

3. The theoretical work of the Harvard Negotiation project produced the still popular work, *Getting to Yes: Negotiating Agreement without Giving In* (Fisher & Ury, 1981).

4. Local community-based mediation centers were founded by counterculture groups, most notably the Community Boards of San Francisco, which continues as a leader in the field.

THE CONTINUUM OF CONFLICT RESOLUTION

How does alternative conflict resolution fit into all the possible ways of resolving conflict? Figure 9.2 shows a continuum of practices/processes. The triangle is divided into thirds. It needs to be conceived as an active volcano and not a static geometrical shape. Conflicts move continually up and down the continuum depending upon their own inner dynamics. Under the volcano's base are all the intense passions and deeply held values and views of the world and self that generate and drive conflict. These drivers are called interests. Interests are most clearly understood as deeply felt violations of a person's or group's sense of safety and wholeness. For example, the elderly widow is angry at her neighbor because he shovels his snow onto her walk. The substantive issue at hand is the snow on her walk. But the underlying interests that are driving the conflict are the violations of long-held values about what a neighbor should do, and of this elderly woman's sense of self-respect and safety, as well as her needs for affiliation, which are being threatened and violated. If

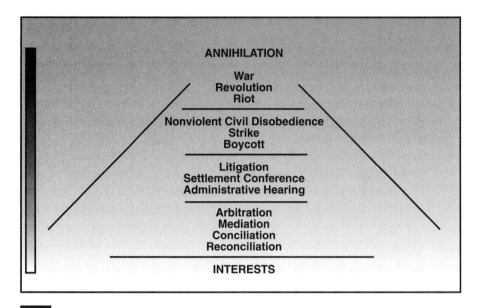

FIGURE 9.2   Continuum of conflict resolution.

these interests are not met, the conflict will escalate and travel up the funnel.

Mediators are fond of saying that issues, the substantive matter of the dispute, are settled through the satisfaction of interests. Interests, for their part, are usually couched in the language of fear, rage, and righteous self-indignation. If conflicts are settled using one of the methods included in the bottom third of the triangle, they have a very good chance of being settled permanently and with optimal healing. It bodes well to try to find appropriate interest-based means of conflict resolution at this level.

If conflicts are not resolved at this bottom level, the pressures keep building until a rights-based method is attempted. These are listed in the middle third of the triangle. People want their "day in court." Our schools and televisions saturate us with this model of resolution. Often, however, there is such an imbalance of power that a person or group is disenfranchised and has no recourse to good legal counsel, or has no way of formulating a lawsuit. In such cases, the conflict escalates and ultimately explodes into either nonviolent or violent modes of expression.

These power-based methods of resolving conflict are included in the top third of the triangle. Frequently weaker parties to a dispute need to attempt a power-based mode to get attention from their adversaries in order to move the conflict into a rights-based or interest-based arena. Because of the complex interplay of interests, rights, and power, persons in conflict never operate at only one point on the continuum. An important principle to note is that disputants increase their control and sense of empowerment over the process and the outcome as they move down the continuum, and, conversely, they experience an increasing loss of empowerment and control over the process and outcomes as they move up the continuum. This is the most cogent reason for encouraging the use of a process as close to the bottom of the continuum as is possible in the circumstances.

THE ROLE OF A NEUTRAL THIRD PARTY

Most conflict resolution methods listed in the interest-based arena need the services of a neutral third party trained in conciliation, mediation, or arbitration.

Conciliation is the assistance of a third party informally helping the disputing parties negotiate a mutually acceptable, interest-based solution to their conflict. The conciliator accomplishes this facilitation as a go-between either in person or by telephone.

Mediation is defined as the use of a formal, voluntary process in which the mediator facilitates settlement negotiations that lead to an informed and mutually acceptable, interest-based settlement. The settlement is written up and, when signed by the parties, can be legally binding.

Arbitration is a forum where disputants, representing themselves, present their sides to the dispute and receive a decision from the arbitrator that is predetermined to be either binding or nonbinding. Arbitration may be voluntary or mandated.

The current reality is that most conflict is settled one way or another by the disputants themselves, unassisted by a third party. Practically all people in conflict have few if any tools to attempt productive resolution. Social and economic dislocation being what it is today, every institution in American society is in distress and producing conflict, evidenced by increasing occurrences of violent outcomes of conflict. In an ideal state, all parents and teachers would have the skills to model, teach, and instill children with the communication skills, problem-solving skills, negotiating skills, and strong sense of self-esteem and self-empowerment that it takes to be part of a dispute and settle it without the need for a third party. Schools are just beginning to offer this kind of training in social and emotional literacy. Training programs in student peer mediation are gaining credibility as a means of giving children life skills and at the same time help inoculate them against the youth culture of drugs and gang violence.

It will take quite a few more generations of parents and teachers to make a big enough impact on positive social change. What do we do until the millennium? In the meantime, there are community-based dispute resolution centers being established throughout the United States and Canada. These dispute resolution services are designed to be easily accessible and affordable. They are often not-for-profit agencies or departments of local governments, staffed either by paid employees or volunteers. In either case, staff at these agencies usually go through extensive training and practical experience before being credentialed as senior mediators.

THE MEDIATION PROCESS

Many types of mediation models are used by mediators in all areas of conflict resolution. Comparing two very different areas of application will demonstrate the wide variety of practice in the field. Labor-management and construction industry conflicts have traditionally used one mediator who alternatively caucuses with all parties, shuttling back and forth in many daylong marathons until disputants are worn down and impasses are broken down. In contrast, many family mediators use comediators who meet with both parties face-to-face and achieve gender balance and safety for couples in high conflict. Whatever the differences in practice, there are some underlying commonalities to the philosophy and practice of mediation in all its forms. In all types of mediation, the mediator is trained to be a neutral facilitator of a specific process. Also, in all types of mediation, there are four discernible phases or functions to the process:

1. Securing process agreements. The mediator asks: Do the disputants agree to enter into mediation voluntarily, to negotiate in good faith, and to abide by rules of common courtesy? Do they understand that mediators will not act as judges, advocates, or attorneys? Do they agree that mediation is a confidential process and that mediators cannot be called to testify in any future litigation of the conflict?

2. Information gathering. Disputants tell their stories while mediators summarize and clarify, trying to ascertain the issues and interests that comprise the conflict.

3. Exploring options for resolutions. Mediators help disputants to work collaboratively to brainstorm and evaluate possible solutions to the conflict.

4. Securing content agreements. Mediators help disputants write out mutually satisfactory agreements in their own words. The process belongs to the disputants. They need to feel safe enough to deal honestly and creatively with each other. Disputants need to be helped to make the process theirs so that the solutions are truly theirs.

When a mediated process is successful, disputants are satisfied in three areas: substantively, psychologically, and procedurally. They have a positive feeling about the resolution of the issues, about themselves and their adversary, and about the fairness and effectiveness of the process.

MEDIATION PROCESS AND THE MODELING AND ROLE-MODELING THEORY

One can readily identify how the mediation process is philosophically resonant with the five aims of intervention (Erickson, Tomlin, & Swain, 1983), which are introduced in chapter 1 of this book and described as follows:

1. Mediation requires that the mediator be the guardian of the process, so that a safe negotiating environment is created and maintained and so that the disputants can build trust in the process. The mediator meets the disputants on their home ground, respecting their view of the world.

2. Mediators promote self-esteem in the disputants by being attentive listeners, by gently reframing disputants' desires and assisting them to assess what is practical and reasonable, and by being disinterestedly interested in offering hope and congratulations when forward movement has been achieved.

3. Mediators facilitate self-empowerment to a great degree by respecting the ability of the disputants to work out their own agreements, by keeping the locus of control regarding the content of the dispute with the disputants, and by helping disputants adhere to a process that when followed, will work in their behalf.

4. Mediators promote a self-awareness of the disputants' inherent strengths and abilities by assisting disputants to problem solve, to systematically generate alternative solutions, and to evaluate possible solutions for suitability of the disputants' interests and values.

5. Mediation and attendant dissolution of stressors promote the most innate drives to health, individuation, and self-actualization by facilitating agreements that have been tested to be in the disputants' mutual best interests.

PRACTICAL APPLICATION FOR NURSES

The Nurse as the Third Party

Before serving as a mediator, nurses must address the following issues:

1. Do you have a conceptual understanding of the role of the neutral person and the process of mediation? Have

you taken any training that prepares you for the behavioral skills needed to mediate successfully?

2. Can you remain impartial? Are you aware of any internal biases and can you set them aside in order to act in an impartial manner so as not to compromise your neutral role?

3. Can you honor confidentiality to a fault so that a safe mediating environment can be created for the disputants?

4. Can your prior relationships with all parties be disclosed to all parties so that their perception of impartiality is upheld?

5. Can you stay within the role of the mediator? Closely helping roles must be set aside for this very distinct role while you are wearing the hat of the third party. While it is eminently helpful and empowering, mediation is not therapy or social work.

6. Is the dispute you are contemplating facilitating open to mediation? This question leads to the next set of guidelines.

Assessing a Conflict Situation for Mediation

To assess a conflict situation for mediation, ask the following questions:

1. Do all parties recognize that a dispute exists?

2. Can all parties that need to be part of a final settlement agreement be involved in the mediation? Another way to ask this is: Do all the people negotiating have the proper authority to enter into written settlement agreements?

3. Do all parties have intellectual and emotional capacities to negotiate in their own best interest and keep agreed-upon settlements?

4. Is there such a disparity in power between the parties that a level playing field cannot be created in the mediation session?

5. Do all parties appear to be on the same timetable regarding their willingness to put down their weapons and voluntarily attempt to mediate? Or does it seem that they will likely use mediation as one more weapon?

6. Do all parties appear to be ready to try to take advantage of the safe and quiet space that you are offering as a mediator to allow them to start to sort out their needs, feelings, and interests?

7. Do all parties appear to be able to envision what a settlement might look like or are they stuck firmly in the past with a rigid bottom line?

Preparing Clients to Consider Mediation

Conciliation is the little understood and rarely honored art of preparing disputants to enter into more formal face-to-face mediation. One could call this phase of mediation intake and case development. Behind the scenes international diplomacy that helps warring parties put down their weapons long enough to consider sitting down around a peace table is a good example of this very important but little researched work. Nurses are in a perfect situation with their clients to deal very effectively with only one party to a dispute. By listening actively and knowing when to begin problem-solving options with their clients, nurses can open up the possibility of mediation and help prepare their clients to be actively engaged disputants in mediation.

In dealing with either one's own strong emotions or in facilitating other persons to deal with their emotions, it is important to keep in mind that problem solving, personal empowerment, negotiation with the opponent, or any other activity that requires higher cerebral functioning is not appropriate until equilibrium can be reestablished or the arousal can be controlled enough so that restimulation is kept to a minimum. The ventilation of strong emotion is the first step in facilitating healthy conflict resolution.

Active Listening for One Party to a Dispute

The most important behavioral tool in helping a client deal with the emotions that conflict inspires is active listening. Active listening has three components. Attending with the appropriate open body position, eye contact, head nods, and nonverbal vocalizations such as "uh huh" lets the speaker know that he is being listened to with respect and attention. Reflecting back to the person both the content and the emotional tone of her message lets the speaker know that she has been heard and understood. Reframing the content of the message gives additional depth to the reflection as well as gives the speaker the opportunity to look at the issues in a new light with the possibility of new insights. The following example illustrates a helping interchange in which no advice is given, no problem solving is attempted, but solely good active listening is engaged by the nurses.

> Client: I'm enraged at the way I've been treated by the clinic staff! They have misplaced records from last year's series of X rays and no one has had the graciousness to even apologize to me. I've never been treated with such rudeness and contempt!

> Nurse: Huh . . . so they've lost some important X-ray records of yours and to add insult to injury you felt badly treated in your dealing with the staff. Is it the records staff you're speaking about?

> Client: Exactly. Oh, I know they're probably overworked and underpaid, but I'm so worried already about this condition, this is just one more little thing I don't need right now. (starting to weep)

> Nurse: Yes, I understand. You're feeling particularly vulnerable right now and this lack of respect you experienced is just the last straw for you.

> Client: It sure is. They're rude and insensitive people! I should talk with their supervisor and lodge a complaint.

> Nurse: So you'd like to let their supervisor know how you feel. Maybe that would make you feel better. If you went and talked to the right person, what else do you need, what else would you have to say? . . .

SUMMARY

Conflict is a common fact of life. It is also a major stressor and contributor to disease processes when it is not dealt with effectively. All cultures have developed processes to manage interpersonal and multiparty conflict. In the past fifteen years, there has been a steady growth in the use of alternative dispute resolution (ADR) methods in North America. Mediation is the most widely used of these. Many institutions are experimenting with ADR. Courts, government, businesses, and communities continue to spread the application of interest-based negotiations with the help of trained mediators. Community-based dispute resolution centers continue to be established throughout North America. Mediation is proving to be efficient and effective in resolving a wide variety of civil disputes. Mediation skills are starting to be taught to students and peer mediation programs are becoming more common in schools.

Mediation is a voluntary, formal process in which a trained neutral person facilitates settlement negotiations leading to a written settlement agreement. It always involves the components of securing process agreements, gathering information, assessing options for settlements, and writing out the settlement agreements.

As helping professionals, nurses are in an ideal position to listen actively when clients are in conflict, assess the appropriateness for mediation, and do the preliminary problem-solving work with clients that prepares them for mediation. Also, nurses can help clients find appropriate community-based mediation resources in their community. In efforts to promote health and peace, knowledge and skill in conflict resolution are important to every nurse.

References

Erickson, H., Tomlin, E., & Swain, M.A. (1983). *Modeling and Role-Modeling: A theory and paradigm for nursing.* Lexington, SC: Pine Press.

Fischer, R., & Ury, W. (1981). *Getting to yes: Negotiated agreement without giving in.* Boston: Houghton Mifflin Company.

INDEX